Study Guide for Understanding Nursing Research

Building an Evidence-Based Practice

5th Edition

Nancy Burns and Susan K. Grove

Study Guide prepared by

Susan K. Grove, PhD, RN, ANP-BC, GNP-BC
Professor of Nursing
College of Nursing
The University of Texas at Arlington
Arlington, Texas

Jennifer Gray, RN, PhD
Associate Professor
Associate Dean and Department Chair
Department of Nursing Administration, Education, and Research Programs
College of Nursing
The University of Texas at Arlington
Arlington, Texas

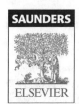

SAUNDERS

ELSEVIER

ELSEVIER
SAUNDERS

3251 Riverport Lane
Maryland Heights, Missouri 63043

Study Guide for Understanding Nursing Research:
Building an Evidence-Based Practice, 5th edition

ISBN: 978-1-4377-1705-1

Notice

Knowledge and best practice in this field are constantly changing. As new research and experience broaden our knowledge, changes in practice, treatment, and drug therapy may become necessary or appropriate. Readers are advised to check the most current information provided (i) on procedures featured or (ii) by the manufacturer of each product to be administered, to verify the recommended dose or formula, the method and duration of administration, and contraindications. It is the responsibility of the practitioner, relying on their own experience and knowledge of the patient, to make diagnoses, to determine dosages and the best treatment for each individual patient, and to take all appropriate safety precautions. To the fullest extent of the law, neither the Publisher nor the authors assume any liability for any injury and/or damage to persons or property arising out of or related to any use of the material contained in this book.

The Publisher

International Standard Book Number: 978-1-4377-1705-1

Acquisitions Editor: Maureen Iannuzzi
Editorial Assistant: Julia Curcio
Publishing Services Manager: Jeffery Patterson
Project Manager: Tracey Schriefer
Design Direction: Karen Pauls

Printed in the United States of America

Last digit is the print number: 9 8 7 6 5 4 3 2

To the nursing students who are our next generation of researchers essential for building an evidence-based practice for nursing.

Susan & Jennifer

To my parents who are so supportive and proud of my publishing activities.

Susan

To my husband, Randy, for supporting my dreams.

Jennifer

We hope that this Study Guide is helpful to you in learning the steps of the research process, critically appraising studies, and synthesizing research findings to facilitate an evidence-based practice for your patients and their families.

Susan K. Grove
Jennifer Gray

Reviewers

Sara Clutter, PhD, RN
Assistant Professor of Nursing
Waynesburg University
Waynesburg, Pennsylvania

Teresa M. O'Neill, RNC, APRN, PhD
Our Lady of Holy Cross College
New Orleans, Louisiana

Nina Ouimette RN-BC, MS, EdD
Patty Hanks Shelton School of Nursing
Abilene, Texas

Jeanne M. Sorrell, PhD, RN, FAAN
Senior Nurse Researcher
Cleveland Clinic
Cleveland, Ohio

Molly J. Walker, PhD, RN, CNS, CNE
Angelo State University
San Angelo, Texas

Fatma A. Youssef, DNSc, MPH, RN
Marymount University
Arlington, Virginia

Preface

The amount of knowledge generated through research is rapidly escalating in nursing. This empirical knowledge is critical for developing an evidence-based practice in nursing that is both high-quality and cost-effective for patients, families, providers, and health care agencies. As a nursing student and registered nurse, you will be encouraged to read, critically appraise, and use research findings to develop protocols, algorithms, and policies for practice. We recognize that learning research terminology and reading and critically appraising research reports are complex and sometimes overwhelming activities. Thus, we have developed this Study Guide to assist you in clarifying, comprehending, analyzing, synthesizing, and applying the content presented in your textbook, *Understanding Nursing Research*, 5th edition.

This edition of the Study Guide is organized according to the steps of the research process and includes exercises that address the revised content on problem, purpose, literature review, framework, ethics, design, sampling, measurement, and statistics. We have expanded the content on qualitative research in the textbook and included a current qualitative research article with two quantitative studies that are critically appraised throughout this Study Guide. The 5th edition of the textbook also includes an extensive expansion of the content on evidence-based practice. You are provided exercises to facilitate your reading of syntheses of research and using this knowledge in developing evidence-based protocols, algorithms, and policies in clinical agencies.

The Study Guide is organized into 14 chapters, which are consistent with the chapters of the textbook. Each chapter presents you with learning exercises that require various levels of knowledge and critical thinking skills. These exercises are organized using the following headings: Key Terms, Key Ideas, Making Connections, Crossword Puzzle, Exercises in Critical Appraisal, and Going Beyond. In some exercises, you will define relevant terms or identify key ideas. In other exercises, you will demonstrate comprehension of the research process by connecting one idea to another. Some exercises are crossword puzzles that will make learning research fun. In the most complex exercises, you will apply your new research knowledge by conducting critical appraisals of published quantitative and qualitative studies.

After completing the exercises for each chapter, you will be able to review the answers in Appendix A and assess your understanding of the content. Based on your correct and incorrect responses, you will be able to focus your study to improve your knowledge of each chapter's content.

Completing the exercises in the Study Guide can provide you with a background for reading, analyzing, and synthesizing the evidence from research reports for application in practice.

How to Get the Most Out of this Study Guide

The exercises in this Study Guide were designed to assist you in comprehending the content in your textbook, conducting critical appraisals of nursing studies, and using research knowledge to promote an evidence-based practice. You will need to read each chapter in your text before completing the chapters in this Study Guide. Scan the entire chapter to get an overall view of the content. Then read the textbook chapter with the intent of increasing your comprehension of each section. As you examine each section, pay careful attention to the terms that are defined. If the meaning of a term is not clear to you, look up its definition in the Glossary and identify other pages focused on the term in the Index at the back of the textbook. Highlight key ideas in each section. Examine tables and figures as they are referenced in the text. Mark sections that you do not sufficiently understand. Jot down questions to ask your instructor in class or privately.

After carefully reading a chapter in the text, use the Study Guide and online questions and exercises (available at http://evolve.elsevier.com/Burns/understanding/) to further enhance your understanding of the research process.

Each chapter in the Study Guide corresponds to its related chapter in your textbook. There are five main sections provided for Study Guide chapters: Key Terms, Key Ideas, Making Connections, Crossword Puzzles, and Exercises in Critical Appraisal, as well as an occasional Going Beyond exercise.

Key Terms

Key terms have been identified for each chapter to assist you in becoming familiar with essential terminology for understanding the research process. Knowing these terms before you attend a class lecture on the content will give you an edge in grasping the lecture content and doing well on course exams. As you read the text, do not skip over terms in the chapter that are unfamiliar to you. Instead, get in the habit of marking unfamiliar words as you read and looking up their definitions in the Glossary at the end of the text.

Key Ideas

This section of the Study Guide identifies important information in each chapter for you. The fill-in-the-blank questions include both short- and long-answer formats and will assist you in identifying essential chapter content that you might have missed. You may need to refer to specific sections of the text to complete some of the questions.

Making Connections

The Making Connections exercises promote linking ideas to facilitate the comprehension, analysis, and synthesis of content related to the research process. Matching questions are frequently used to assist you in performing these critical thinking skills.

Crossword Puzzles

The Crossword Puzzle section is designed for having fun while learning the research process. These were developed to help you increase your familiarity with the terms used in the chapter.

Exercises in Critical Appraisal

Critical appraisal exercises are provided to give you experiences in critically appraising published studies. In some cases, brief quotes are provided, with questions addressing information specific to the chapter content. The majority of the critical appraisal exercises focus on the three published studies that are provided in Appendix B of this Study Guide. Two of the studies are quantitative and one of the studies is qualitative so you can have experience in critically appraising both types of studies. The quantitative studies include one correlational and one quasi-experimental type of study. On completing the Study Guide, you can incorporate the critical appraisal information you have learned to perform an overall critical appraisal of these three studies. In addition, you can take the knowledge you have learned and apply it in the critical appraisal of other published quantitative and qualitative studies.

Going Beyond

Occasionally exercises have been included that provide suggestions for further study. You might use these activities to test your new knowledge. If the content of a particular chapter interests you, this section might direct you in learning more about that step of the research process.

Answers

The answers to all Study Guide questions are provided in Appendix A in the back of the Study Guide. However, we recommend that you not refer to these answers except to check your own responses to the questions. You will learn more by reading the textbook and searching for the answers on your own.

Published Studies

Reprints of three published studies are provided in Appendix B. These studies are referenced in many of the questions throughout the Study Guide. Two additional published studies referenced in the Study Guide are found in the Research Articles section of the online resources.

You are now ready to begin your adventure of learning about the research process to build an evidence-based practice.

Contents

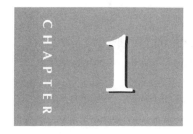

CHAPTER 1

Introduction to Nursing Research and Evidence-Based Practice

INTRODUCTION

You need to read Chapter 1 and then complete the following exercises. These exercises will assist you in learning key research terms, identifying the types of research conducted in nursing, and understanding evidence-based practice. The answers to these exercises are in Appendix A under Chapter 1.

KEY TERMS

Acquiring Knowledge and Research Methods

Directions: Match each term below with its correct definition. Each term is used only once and all terms are defined.

a. Borrowing
b. Deductive reasoning
c. Description
d. Explanation
e. Inductive reasoning
f. Intuition
g. Knowledge
h. Nursing research

i. Outcomes research
j. Personal experience
k. Prediction
l. Qualitative research
m. Quantitative research
n. Reasoning
o. Role modeling

Definitions

_G_ 1.   Information acquired in a variety of ways that is expected to be an accurate reflection of reality and is used to guide practice.

_H_ 2.   A scientific process that validates and refines existing knowledge and generates new knowledge that directly and indirectly influences nursing practice.

_E_ 3.   Reasoning from the specific to the general.

_J_ 4.   Gaining knowledge by being personally involved in a situation, such as providing care to patients in ICU.

_M_ 5.   A formal, objective, systematic research process to describe, test relationships, or examine cause-and-effect interactions among variables.

_B_ 6.   Reasoning from the general to the specific or from a general premise to a particular situation.

_C_ 7.   Knowledge generated from research that includes evidence for identifying and understanding the nature of nursing phenomena for practice.

_F_ 8.   Insight or understanding of a situation or event as a whole that usually cannot be logically explained.

_L_ 9.   A systematic, subjective research approach used to describe life experiences and give them meaning.

_D_ 10. Knowledge generated from research that clarifies relationships among variables.

___ 11.   An important scientific methodology that was developed to examine the end results of patient care.

___ 12.   Knowledge generated from research that enables one to estimate the probability of a specific outcome in a given situation.

___ 13.   The appropriation and use of knowledge from other fields or disciplines to guide nursing practice.

___ 14.   Learning by imitating the behaviors of an expert and the process of teaching less-experienced professionals by demonstrating model behaviors.

___ 15.   Processing and organizing ideas to reach conclusions and examples include problematic and logistics.

Evidence-Based Practice Terms

Directions: Match each term with the correct definition.

a.   Best research evidence
b.   Clinical expertise
c.   Critical appraisal of research
d.   Evidence-based guidelines
e.   Evidence-based practice

Definitions

___ 1.   The conscientious integration of best research evidence with clinical expertise and patient values and needs in the delivery of high-quality, cost-effective health care.

___ 2.   Knowledge and skills of the health care professional providing care and is determined for a nurse by years of clinical experience, current knowledge of the research and clinical literature, and educational preparation.

___ 3.   The strongest empirical knowledge available generated from the synthesis of quality study findings to address a practice problem.

___ 4.   Rigorous explicit clinical guidelines developed based on the best research evidence available in that area.

___ 5.   Careful examination of all aspects of a study to judge its strengths, limitations, meaning, and significance.

Processes Used to Synthesize Research Evidence

Directions: Match each term with the correct definition.

a.   Integrative review
b.   Meta-analysis
c.   Metasummary
d.   Metasynthesis
e.   Systematic review

Definitions

___ 1.   Structured, comprehensive synthesis of quantitative and outcomes studies and meta-analyses in a particular health care area to determine the best research evidence available for expert clinicians to use to promote evidence-based practice.

___ 2.   Process for synthesizing qualitative research findings to sum the findings across reports in a target area.

___ 3.   The identification, analysis, and synthesis of research findings from independent quantitative, outcomes, and qualitative studies to determine the current knowledge in a particular area.

_B_ 4. Qualitative synthesis technique that provides a fully integrated novel description or explanation of a target event or experience versus a summary of that event.

_D_ 5. A type of study and research synthesis that statistically pools the results from previous studies into a single quantitative analysis and provides one of the highest levels of evidence for an intervention's efficacy.

KEY IDEAS

How Research Influences Practice

Directions: The knowledge generated through research is essential to provide a scientific basis for the description, explanation, prediction, and control of nursing practice. Write a definition and provide an example of these four terms.

1. Description: identifying the nature & attributes of nursing phenomena descriptive knowledge generated through Research

   Example: who are at risk for HIV

2. Explanation: Clarifying relationship among variables

   Example: Devloping Pressure ulcere

3. Prediction: Estimating the probability of a specific outcome

   Example: effect of nutrition w/ obese children

4. Control: *abulity to manipulate a situation to produce a desired outcome*

    _____

    _____

    Example: *Back massages on relief of arthritic pain*

    _____

    _____

Historical Events Influencing Nursing Research

Directions: Fill in the blanks in this section with the appropriate word(s) or numbers.

1. ___*Nightingale*___ is considered the first nurse researcher.

2. The journal *Nursing Research* was first published in ___*1952*___.

3. Many national and international research conferences have been sponsored by _____ *Sigma Theta Tau*, the International Honor Society for Nursing to communicate study findings.

4. Identify three nursing research journals that were first published from 1979 to 1988.

    a. *Research in Nursing & Health*

    b. *Western Journal of Nursing Research*

    c. *Applied Nursing Research*

5. The *Annual Review of Nursing Research* includes *integrative reviews of research* ___*Valle*___.

6. The National Center for Nursing Research (NCNR) was established in ___*1985*___ by the National Institutes of Health.

7. The NCNR is now called the *National Institute for Nursing Research*

8. The purpose of the National Institute for Nursing Research (NINR) is ___*conduct*___, ___*support*___, and ___*dissemination of information*___ regarding basic and clinical nursing research.

9. Identify the mission of the NINR for the 21st century. *promote & improve the health of individuals, families communities*

    _____

    _____

10. The focus of nursing research from the 1980s to the present is the conduct of _Clinical_ research.

11. _Agency for Health Care Policy & Research_ was established in 1989 to facilitate the conduct of outcomes research and the communication of the findings to health care provider.

12. The Agency for Health Care Policy and Research (AHCPR) was renamed in 1999 and became the _Agency for Healthcare Research & Quality_. This agency is playing a major role in the development of evidence-based guidelines for use in practice.

13. The Agency for Healthcare Research and Quality has an excellent website that includes evidence-based practice guidelines at _guidelines.gov_.

14. The Department of Health and Human Services (DHHS) increased the visibility of and identified priorities for health-promotion research by publishing _Healthy People 2010_.

15. The type of research that is focused on the quality and cost-effectiveness of health care, which increased in the 1990s and will continue to expand in the 21st century, is _Outcomes Research_.

Acquiring Knowledge in Nursing

Directions: Fill in the blanks with the appropriate responses.

1. List five ways of acquiring knowledge in nursing, and provide an example of each.

   a. _Tradition → giving report on hospitalized patient_

   b. _Authority → expert nurse, education_

   c. _Borrowing → using other knowlege_

   d. _Trial & Error → trying interventions like sleep at night_

   e. _Research → qualitative, quantitative, & outcomes research method_

2. Benner's 1984 book, *From Novice to Expert: Excellence and Power in Clinical Practice*, describes the importance of _personal experience_ in acquiring nursing knowledge.

3. Identify Benner's five levels of experience in the development of clinical knowledge and expertise.

   a. _novice_

   b. _advance beginner_

   c. _competent_

   d. _proficient_

   e. _expert_

4. _Research, Empirical, Scientific_ knowledge provides an evidence base for the description, explanation, prediction, and control of nursing practice.

5. A "gut feeling" or "hunch" is an example of _____intuition_____, which nurses have found useful in identifying patients' serious problems.

6. _____Tradition_____ are knowledge based on customs and past trends, such as providing hospitalized patients a bath every morning.

7. What type of reasoning is used in the following example? _____deductive Reasoning_____

   Human beings experience pain.
   Babies are human beings.
   Therefore, babies experience pain.

8. Identify four important outcomes that might be examined with outcomes research.

   a. _____patient health status_____
   b. _____patient satisfaction_____
   c. _____quality of care_____
   d. _____provider satisfaction_____

MAKING CONNECTIONS

Linking Research Methods to Types of Research

Directions: Match the following research methods with the specific type of research.

Research Methods

a. Qualitative research method
b. Quantitative research method

Types of Research

_b_ 1. Correlational research
_b_ 2. Descriptive research
_a_ 3. Ethnographic research
_b_ 4. Experimental research
_a_ 5. Grounded theory research
_a_ 6. Historical research
_a_ 7. Phenomenological research
_b_ 8. Quasi-experimental research

Determining the Strength of Levels of Research Evidence

Directions: List the following examples of research evidence in order from the strongest or best research evidence to the weakest research evidence. The strongest research evidence should be a 1 and the weakest research evidence should be a 6.

_4_ Single correlational study examining the relationships of body mass index, hours watching television per week, and hours on the computer each day.

_1_ Systematic review used to develop the evidence-based guidelines for diagnosis and management of hypertension.

__3__ Integrative review of correlational and descriptive studies about H1N1 flu.

__2__ Meta-analysis of experimental studies (randomized clinical trials [RCT]) and quasi-experimental studies to examine interventions to reduce the weight of obese school-age children.

__6__ Opinions of respected authorities on the management of diabetes.

__5__ Single qualitative study of the process of weaning older adult patients from mechanical ventilation.

Nurses' Roles in Research

Directions: Match the levels of nurses' educational preparation with the research activities that each group of nurses is primarily responsible for according to the guidelines of the American Nurses Association (ANA).

Nurses' Educational Preparation

a. Bachelor of Science in Nursing (BSN)

b. Master of Science in Nursing (MSN)

c. Doctorate of Nursing Practice (DNP)

d. Doctorate of Philosophy (PhD) in Nursing

e. Postdoctorate

Research Activities

__A__ 1. Uses research evidence in practice with guidance

__E__ 2. Develops and coordinates funded research programs

__A,B__ 3. Critically appraises studies

__P,E__ 4. Develops nursing knowledge through research and theory development

__C__ 5. Participates in the development of evidence-based guidelines

__B,C__ 6. Collaborates in conducting research projects

__D__ 7. Conducts independent research projects

__E__ 8. Critically appraises studies and synthesizes research evidence to develop and refine protocols and policies for a selected health care agency

__E__ 9. Mentors PhD prepared researchers

__D&E__ 10. Coordinates research teams of BSN-, MSN-, and DNP-prepared nurses

EXERCISES IN CRITICAL APPRAISAL

Directions: Locate the research articles (listed below) in Appendix B. Review the titles, abstracts, and authors' credentials for these three articles. Identify the type of research conducted in each study.

Research Methods

a. Outcomes research method

b. Qualitative research method

c. Quantitative research method

__C__ 1. Bindler, R. C., Massey, L. K., Shultz, J. A., Mills, P. E., & Short, R. (2007). Metabolic syndrome in a multiethnic sample of school children: Implications for the pediatric nurse (provided in Appendix B).

__C__ 2. Padula, C. A., Yeaw, E., & Mistry, S. (2009). A home-based nurse-coached inspiratory muscle training intervention in heart failure (provided in Appendix B).

__B__ 3. Schachman, K. A. (2010). Online fathering: The experience of first-time fatherhood in combat-deployed troops (provided in Appendix B).

Researchers' Credentials

Directions: Review the educational, research, and clinical credentials of the authors of the three research articles in Appendix B. The articles include some information about the authors, but you can also search for the authors' credentials online.

1. Discuss whether or not Bindler et al. (2007) have the educational, research, and clinical preparation to conduct their study.

    _____

    _____

    _____

    _____

    _____

    _____

    _____

    _____

    _____

    _____

2. Discuss whether or not Padula et al. (2009) have the educational, research, and clinical preparation to conduct their study.

    _____

    _____

    _____

    _____

    _____

    _____

    _____

    _____

    _____

    _____

    _____

3. Discuss whether or not Schachman (2010) has the educational, research, and clinical preparation to conduct her study.

_____

_____

_____

_____

_____

_____

_____

_____

_____

_____

GOING BEYOND

Directions: Post your ideas for the following on your Research Course website. Look for input from other students and faculty.

Your critical appraisal of the title for the Padula et al. (2009) article. The title was: A home-based nurse-coached inspiratory muscle training intervention in heart failure.

_____

_____

_____

_____

_____

_____

_____

_____

_____

Critically appraise the abstract for the Bindler et al. (2007) study.

_____

_____

_____

_____

_____

_____

_____

_____

_____

_____

2

Introduction to the Quantitative Research Process

INTRODUCTION

You need to read Chapter 2 and then complete the following exercises. These exercises will assist you in learning the steps of the quantitative research process; identifying the different types of quantitative research (descriptive, correlational, quasi-experimental, and experimental); and reading research reports. The answers for the following exercises are in Appendix A under Chapter 2.

KEY TERMS

Directions: Match each term below with its correct definition. Each term is used only once and all terms are defined.

a. Applied research
b. Assumptions
c. Basic research
d. Control
e. Correlational research
f. Descriptive research
g. Design
h. Framework
i. Generalization
j. Interpretation of research outcomes

k. Methodological limitations
l. Pilot study
m. Quantitative research process
n. Quasi-experimental research
o. Reading research reports
p. Research problem
q. Research purpose
r. Sampling
s. Setting
t. Theoretical limitations

Definitions

__m__ 1. Formal, objective, systematic process to describe, test relationships, and examine cause-and-effect interactions among variables.

__s__ 2. Location for conducting research that can be natural, partially controlled, or highly controlled.

__a__ 3. Scientific investigations conducted to generate knowledge that will directly influence clinical practice.

__d__ 4. Imposing of rules by the researcher to decrease the possibility of error and increase the probability that the study's findings are an accurate reflection of reality.

__r__ 5. Process of selecting a group of people, events, behaviors, or other elements that are representative of the population being studied.

__c__ 6. Scientific investigations for the pursuit of "knowledge for knowledge's sake," or for the pleasure of learning.

__i__ 7. Extension of the implications of the findings from the sample that was studied to the larger population.

l 8. Smaller version of a proposed study conducted to develop and/or refine the methodology, such as the treatment or intervention, measurement instruments, or data collection process to be used in the larger study.

Q 9. The specific goal or focus of a study that directs the remaining steps of the research process.

t 10. The limitations that restrict the abstract generalization of the findings and are reflected in the study framework and the conceptual and operational definitions of the variables.

N 11. Type of quantitative research that is conducted to examine causal relationships or to determine the effect of an independent variable on the dependent variable but lacks the control of an experimental study.

o 12. Use of the skills of skimming, comprehending, and analyzing content from research reports.

f 13. Type of quantitative research that involves the exploration and description of phenomena in real-life situations.

k 14. Limitations, such as a small sample size or poor measurement methods that decrease the credibility of the findings and restrict the population to which the findings can be generalized.

h 15. The abstract, theoretical basis for a study that enables the researcher to link the findings to nursing's body of knowledge.

g 16. Blueprint for the conduct of a study that maximizes control over factors that could interfere with the study's desired outcome.

e 17. Type of quantitative research that involves the systematic investigation of relationships between or among variables.

J 18. Step in the research process that involves examining the results of data analysis, forming conclusions, considering implications for nursing, exploring the significance of the findings, generalizing the findings, and suggesting further studies.

P 19. A step in the research process that identifies the gap in nursing knowledge needed for practice and indicates an area for further research.

b 20. Statements that are taken for granted or are considered true even though they have not been scientifically tested.

KEY IDEAS

Control in Quantitative Research

Directions: Fill in the blanks with the appropriate word(s).

1. An experimental study is conducted in a(n) _highly controlled_ setting.

2. Extraneous variables need to be controlled in _quasi-experimental_ and _experimental_ _____ types of quantitative research to ensure that the findings are accurate reflections of reality.

3. _descriptive_ and _correlational_ studies are usually uncontrolled by the researcher and conducted in natural settings.

4. _experimental_ studies need to include random selection of the study sample.

5. Frequently, a(n) _nonRandom/nonprob_ sampling method is used in descriptive and correlational studies. However, a(n) _Random/prob_ sampling method might also be used.

6. A subject's home is an example of a(n) _natural_ setting.

7. Laboratories and research centers are examples of _highly controlled_ settings.

8. Researcher control is greatest in what type of quantitative research? _experimental_

9. Hospital units are examples of _partially controlled_ settings that allow the researcher to control some of the extraneous variables.

Steps of the Research Process

Directions: Fill in the blanks with the appropriate word(s).

1. The research process is similar to the _problem solving_ and the _nursing_ processes.

2. List the steps of the quantitative research process in their order of occurrence.

    Step 1 _Research problem_

    Step 2 _literature Review_

    Step 3 _Study framework_

    Step 4 _Research objectives_

    Step 5 _study variables_

    Step 6 _assumptions_

    Step 7 _limitations_

    Step 8 _research design_

    Step 9 _population & sample_

    Step 10 _methods & measurements_

    Step 11 _data collection_

    Step 12 _data analysis_

    Step 13 _research outcomes_

3. Assumptions are _statements seen as true even though they need scientifically tested_

4. Identify three common assumptions on which nursing studies have been based.

    a. _People want to assume control_

    b. _stress should be avoided_

    c. _attitudes can be measured w/ a scale_

5. The two types of limitations that might exist in a study are _theoretical_ and _____ _methodological_ .

6. Identify five possible examples of limitations that you might find in published studies.

   a. _weak conceptual def. variables_

   b. _poorly developed framework_

   c. _unclear links_

   d. _small sample size_

   e. _limited control data_

7. A pilot study is _smaller version of a proposed study_

   _____ .

8. Identify four reasons for conducting a pilot study.

   a. _Refine Research treatment_

   b. _identify problems with design_

   c. _try out data analysis_

   d. _identify problems with design_

Reading Research Reports

1. The most common sources for nursing research reports are professional journals. Identify three nursing research journals.

   a. _Advances in Nursing Scien_

   b. _Applied Nursing Research_

   c. _Nursing Research_

2. Identify two clinical journals that include several research articles in each issue.

   a. _Birth_

   b. _Public Health Nursing_

3. Identify the four major sections of a research report.

   a. _introduction_

   b. _method_

   c. _Results_

   d. _Discussion_

4. The methods section of a research report describes how a study was conducted and usually includes:

   a. design

   b. sample

   c. setting

   d. methods of measurement

   e. data collection process

5. The discussion section ties the other sections of the research report together and gives them meaning. This section includes:

   a. major findings

   b. conclusions

   c. limitations

   d. implication

   e. reccommendation

6. The problem and purpose are often identified in which section of a research report? _____

   introduction process

7. The reference list at the end of the article includes all the ___theories___ and ___studies___ _____ that provide bases for the study and are cited in the article.

8. Reading a research report involves ___skimming___, ___comprehending___ _____, and ___analyzing___ the content of the report.

9. In reading a research report, the comprehending step involves ___comprehending steps___

   _____.

10. In reading a research report, the analyzing step determing value of the researchs reports _____.

MAKING CONNECTIONS

Types of Quantitative Research

Directions: Match the type of quantitative research listed below with the examples of study titles.

a. Descriptive research
b. Correlational research
c. Quasi-experimental research
d. Experimental research

___C___ 1. Determining the effect of a relaxation technique on patients' postoperative pain and anxiety levels.

___A___ 2. Identifying the incidence of HIV in adolescents and young adults.

___B___ 3. Examining the relationships among age, gender, knowledge of AIDS, and use of condoms by college students.

___A___ 4. Describing the coping strategies of chronically ill men and women.

___D___ 5. Determining the effects of position on sacral and heel pressures in hospitalized older adults.

___D___ 6. Determining the effect of impaired physical mobility on skeletal muscle atrophy in laboratory rats.

___A___ 7. Identifying current nursing practice behaviors for male and female nurses working in an intensive care area.

___B___ 8. Examining the relationships among intensive care unit (ICU) stress, anxiety, and recovery rate for patients following cardiac surgery.

___C___ 9. Examining the effects of a preadmission self-instruction program on patients' postoperative activity levels, anxiety levels, pain perception, lengths of hospital stay, and time until return to work.

___D___ 10. Examining the effects of thermal applications on the abdominal temperatures of laboratory dogs.

___B___ 11. Examining the relationships among hardiness, depression, and coping in institutionalized older adults.

___A___ 12. Determining the incidence of drug abuse in registered nurses in community and hospital settings.

___C___ 13. Examining the effect of warm and cold applications on the resolution of IV infiltrations in hospitalized patients.

___A___ 14. Determining the stress levels and desired support of family caregivers of older adults with Alzheimer's disease.

___C___ 15. Examining the effectiveness of breast cancer screening programs for women residing in rural areas.

___A___ 16. Comparing the ages and coping skills of mothers pregnant with the first child in three ethnic groups (Caucasian, African American, and Hispanic).

___B___ 17. Using age, nutritional intake, mobility level, weight, level of cognitive function, and serum albumin to predict the risk for pressure ulcers in hospitalized patients on a medical-surgical unit.

___A___ 18. Describing the severity of fatigue and anxiety in individuals with chronic obstructive pulmonary disease.

___A___ 19. Comparing and contrasting the health-promotion and illness-prevention behaviors of African-American and Caucasian older adults.

___B___ 20. Examining the relationships among the lipid values, blood pressure, weight, and stress levels of adolescents.

CROSSWORD PUZZLE

Directions: Complete the crossword puzzle below. Note that if the answer is more than one word, no blank spaces are left between the words.

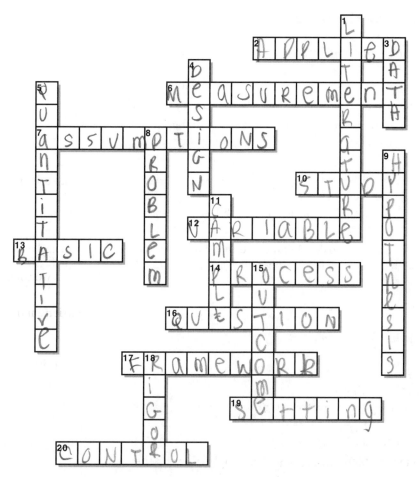

Across

2. Research in which findings are directly useful in practice is _____ research
6. _____ of dependent variables in research
7. Known truths
10. Research project
12. Study treatment is an independent _____
13. Type of research that seeks knowledge for knowledge's sake
14. Nursing _____ to direct nursing care
16. Directs a study
17. Crisis theory could be a study _____
19. Location of research
20. Researchers _____ extraneous variables in a study, if possible

Down

1. What is reviewed prior to conducting a study
3. What is collected in a study
4. Study blueprint
5. Type of nursing research
8. Gap in nursing knowledge for practice
9. Null _____
11. Subjects comprise this
15. Research finding
18. Strict adherence to research plan

EXERCISES IN CRITICAL APPRAISAL

Directions: Read the research articles in Appendix B and answer the following questions.

Type of Quantitative or Qualitative Research

Identify the type of quantitative or qualitative research conducted in each study.

a. Descriptive research
b. Correlational research
c. Quasi-experimental research
d. Experimental research

e. Phenomenological research
f. Grounded theory research
g. Ethnographic research
h. Historical research

_B_ 1. Bindler, R. C., Massey, L. K., Shultz, J. A., Mills, P. E., & Short, R. (2007). Metabolic syndrome in a multiethnic sample of school children: Implications for the pediatric nurse (provided in Appendix B).

_C_ 2. Padula, C. A., Yeaw, E., & Mistry, S. (2009). A home-based nurse-coached inspiratory muscle training intervention in heart failure (provided in Appendix B).

_E_ 3. Schachman, K. A. (2010). Online fathering: The experience of first-time fatherhood in combat-deployed troops (provided in Appendix B).

Type of Setting

Identify the type of setting for each study.

a. Natural setting
b. Partially controlled setting
c. Highly controlled setting

_B_ 4. Bindler et al. (2007) study setting
_A_ 5. Padula et al. (2009) study setting
_A_ 6. Schachman (2010) study setting

Type of Research Conducted (Applied or Basic)

Indicate the type of nursing research conducted in each study.

a. Applied nursing research
b. Basic nursing research

_A_ 7. Bindler et al. (2007) study
_A_ 8. Padula et al. (2009) study
_A_ 9. Schachman (2010) study

3

Introduction to the Qualitative Research Process

INTRODUCTION

You need to read Chapter 3 and then complete the following exercises. These exercises will assist you in learning key terms and reading and comprehending published qualitative studies. The answers for the following exercises are in Appendix A under Chapter 3.

KEY TERMS

Directions: Match each term below with its correct definition. Each term is used only once and all terms are defined.

a. Historical research
b. Qualitative research
c. Transcription
d. Open-ended interview
e. Snowballing
f. Phenomenological research
g. Grounded theory research
h. Gestalt

i. Emic approach
j. Rigor
k. Participant
l. Ethnographic research
m. Field notes
n. Bracketing
o. Secondary source
p. Reflexive thought

Definitions

D 1. Questioning research participants orally without a fixed list of questions.
C 2. Typing a verbatim narrative from a recorded interview or focus group.
J 3. Characteristics of a study that give its findings credibility and greater value.
K 4. A person from whom data are collected during a qualitative study.
N 5. Setting aside one's values and perspectives during the data collecting and analysis process.
O 6. Account of an event by a person who learned about the event from another person.
P 7. Researcher explores personal feelings and experiences that may influence the study and integrates this understanding into the study.
B 8. Systematic, subjective approach to describe life experiences and give them meaning.
F 9. Focused on the lived experience.
e 10. Persons who have provided data for a study tell other eligible persons about the study.
m 11. Notes from a research observation.
i 12. Studying behavior from within a culture.
G 13. Qualitative method that describes social processes and proposes a framework of related concepts.
A 14. Research about from where nursing has come.
H 15. Knowledge about a particular phenomenon is organized into a cluster of linked ideas.
L 16. Study that explores the culture of a specific group of people or an organization.

KEY PERSONS

Directions: Match each person below with the correct description. Each name is used only once and all persons are described.

a.   Philosopher associated with the interpretive approach to phenomenology.

b.   Developed the Sunshine Model of Transcultural Nursing Care.

c.   Nurse who developed mass disaster preparations during the Cold War era.

d.   Philosopher associated with the descriptive approach to phenomenology.

e.   Person who developed the symbolic interaction theory.

f.   Early studies on dying led to the grounded theory method.

_b_ 17.   Leininger

_f_ 18.   Glaser and Strauss

_d_ 19.   Husserl

_a_ 20.   Heidegger

_e_ 21.   Mead

_c_ 22.   Werley

Directions: Define the following terms in your own words without looking at your textbook. Then check your definitions with those in the glossary of your textbook. Using this strategy, you can identify elements of the term that are not yet clear in your mind. Reread that section of the chapter to clarify your understanding of the term.

23. Observation: _Gathering data 1st hand_

24. Coding: _Labeling words & phrases_

25. Historical research: _Study of the past_

26. Researcher-participant relationship: _open & honest communicatn_

KEY IDEAS

Directions: Fill in the blanks with the appropriate word(s).

1.   One premise of qualitative research is that inquiry is _value laden / subjective_.

2.   Qualitative approaches recognize that experiences are unique to the _Individual_.

3.   Symbolic interaction theory explores how persons define _reality_ and how their _beliefs_ affect their actions.

4.   Reading and rereading the data in qualitative research is called being _immersed_ in the data.

5. An ethnographer who goes ___native___ becomes part of the culture and loses objectivity.

6. Interviews that are conducted with open-ended questions and probes would be called ___unstructured___.

7. The person who conducts a focus group and ensures that all participants have the opportunity to speak is called the ___facilitator___.

8. During an observation, the researcher may write ___field notes___ to record what is seen and heard.

9. The sampling method in which a participant recruits another participant is called ___network___.

10. A study investigating the lived experience of a group of women who have sickle cell anemia uses ___phenomenology___ as its research method.

11. ___Heidegger___ is the philosopher whose work is the basis for hermeneutics.

12. Grounded theory was developed by scholars from the discipline of ___sociology___.

13. The description and analysis of a single unit within a real life environment is a(n) ___case study___.

14. ___ethnography___ is the study of the traditions and customs of people.

15. A ___first-hand___ source was written by the person who witnessed the events.

16. Rather than probability sampling in quantitative methodology, qualitative research includes ___nonprobability___ and most often purposive sampling.

17. ___interviews___ include asking participants questions to answer verbally.

18. A computer can help a researcher to ___organize___, ___code___, and ___retrieve___ qualitative data.

19. ___culture___ includes the traditions, language, and customs of a particular group of people.

20. A researcher who wants to understand the causes and context of past events would use ___historical research___.

MAKING CONNECTIONS

Comparing Qualitative and Quantitative Research Methodologies

Directions: Qualitative and quantitative research methods look at research in different ways. For the phrases below, indicate which refer to qualitative methods (QL) and which refer to quantitative methods (QN).

___QN___ 1. Produces "hard" science.

___QN___ 2. Focuses on the analysis of words.

___QL___ 3. Truth is absolute.

QN 4.   Is reductionistic.

QL 5.   Is holistic.

QL 6.   Research findings are considered subjective.

QL 7.   Truth is dynamic.

QN 8.   Control is important.

QN 9.   Objectivity is essential.

QN 10.   Involves the analysis of numbers.

Approaches to Qualitative Research

Directions: Match each qualitative method with its characteristics. Label them a P, G, E, and/or H, according to the key below for each area. Mark all that apply for each type.

P = Phenomenological   E = Ethnographic

G = Grounded theory   H = Historical

E 1.   Studies cultures.

G 2.   Studies social processes.

E 3.   May use key informants.

P 4.   Refers to a philosophy and a research method.

E 5.   Emerged from the discipline of anthropology.

H 6.   Studies the past.

P 7.   Studies the meaning of a lived experience.

G 8.   Seeks to develop a framework of concepts or theory.

H 9.   Develops an inventory of sources.

G 10.   May move from description to discovery and emergent modes.

CROSSWORD PUZZLE

Directions: Complete the crossword puzzle below. Note: If the answer is more than one word, no blank spaces are left between the words.

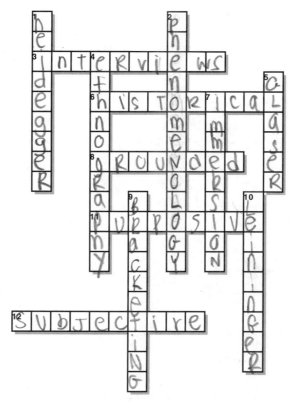

Across

3. Verbal interactions to collect data
6. The study of the past
8. Theory that emerges from the analysis of social processes
11. Selecting participants because of their experiences
12. Personal perspective on an experience

Down

1. Thought leader of interpretive phenomenology
2. Description and analysis of the lived experience
4. It is all about culture
5. Early researcher who developed grounded theory methods
7. Reading, rereading, and reflecting on data
9. Setting aside personal values
10. Mother of ethnonursing

EXERCISES IN CRITICAL APPRAISAL

Directions: Read the Schachman (2010) article in Appendix B of this study guide. Answer the following questions about that qualitative study.

1. What was the purpose of Schachman's study? _____

_____

_____

_____

_____

2. Which qualitative method was used for the study? What rationale was given for using this method?

_____

_____

_____

_____

_____

_____

3. How were the participants recruited for the study? What type of sampling was used?_____

_____

_____

_____

_____

_____

4. Describe the data collection process for the Schachman (2010) study. _____

_____

_____

_____

_____

_____

_____

_____

_____

_____

_____

5. Researchers may use bracketing as part of their study methods. List two strategies used for bracketing.

_____

_____

_____

_____

_____

_____

6. Summarize the theme clusters by completing the following table. Add Main Theme II and the five theme clusters under the appropriate main theme.

Main Theme I: Disruption of the Protector and Provider Role	Main Theme II: _____
Lost Opportunity	

7. Which quotation from a participant was most meaningful to you? Provide a rationale for your choice.

_____

_____

_____

_____

_____

_____

8. Did Schachman (2010) identify limitations of her study? If so, what were those limitations? _____

_____

_____

_____

_____

_____

_____

_____

_____

_____

9. In the discussion, Schachman (2010) included findings about the use of doulas during labor. What gap did she identify that might lead to a future study?

_____

_____

_____

10. What implications for practice did Schachman (2010) recommend? _____

_____

_____

_____

_____

_____

_____

_____

_____

_____

GOING BEYOND

1. Select a qualitative study from a recent nursing journal and complete the following.
   a. Identify the type of qualitative study performed.
   b. Identify the data collection methods used.
   c. Describe how the data were analyzed.
   d. What was done to maintain the quality of the work?
   e. Did the implications for nursing practice fit the study findings?

2. Select one topic in nursing practice that would be appropriate for a qualitative study. Why would a qualitative study be appropriate? How would you approach the research? Share your ideas with your instructor.

4 Examining Ethics in Nursing Research

INTRODUCTION

You need to read Chapter 4 and then complete the following exercises. These exercises will assist you in understanding the ethical aspects of a variety of nursing studies. The answers for these exercises are in Appendix A under Chapter 4.

KEY TERMS

Directions: Match each term below with its correct definition. Each term is used only once and all terms are defined.

a. Anonymity
b. Autonomous agent
c. Benefit-risk ratio
d. Confidentiality
e. Discomfort and harm risks
f. Ethical principles
g. Human rights
h. Individually identifiable health information

i. Informed consent
j. Institutional review
k. Nontherapeutic research
l. Plagiarism
m. Privacy Act
n. Research misconduct
o. Therapeutic research

Definitions

_____ 1. Claims and demands that have been justified in the eyes of an individual or the consensus of a group of individuals and are protected in research.

_____ 2. Condition in which a subject's identity cannot be linked, even by the researcher, with his or her individual responses.

_____ 3. Agreement by a prospective subject to participate voluntarily in a study after he or she has indicated understanding of the essential information about the study.

_____ 4. Research conducted to generate knowledge for a discipline; the results might benefit future patients but will probably not benefit the research subjects.

_____ 5. Process of examining studies for ethical concerns by a committee of peers.

_____ 6. Phrase used to describe the degrees of risk subjects might experience while participating in research. These levels of risk include no anticipated effects, temporary discomfort, unusual levels of temporary discomfort, risk of permanent damage, or certainty of permanent damage.

_____ 7. Freedom of an individual to determine the time, extent, and general circumstances under which private information will be shared with or withheld from others.

_____ 8. Ratio considered by researchers and reviewers of research as they weigh potential benefits and risks in a study to promote the conduct of ethical research.

_____ 9. Research that provides a patient with an opportunity to receive an experimental treatment that might have beneficial results.

____ 10. Principles of respect for persons, beneficence, and justice that are relevant to the conduct of research.

____ 11. Management of private data in research in such a way that subjects' identities are not linked with their responses.

____ 12. Practices such as fabrication, falsification, or forging of data; dishonest manipulation of the study design or methods; and plagiarism.

____ 13. Any information, including demographic information, collected from an individual that is created or received by health care providers, health plan, or health care clearinghouse.

____ 14. Humans who have the freedom to conduct their lives as they choose, without external controls.

____ 15. The appropriation of another person's ideas, processes, results, or words without giving appropriate credit, including those obtained through confidential review of others' research proposal and manuscripts.

KEY IDEAS

Directions: Fill in the blanks with the correct responses.

1. List the elements of informed consent.

   a. _____

   b. _____

   c. _____

   d. _____

2. Identify the types of information that must be included in a study consent form.

   a. _____

   b. _____

   c. _____

   d. _____

   e. _____

   f. _____

   g. _____

   h. _____

   i. _____

   j. _____

3. _____ consent means that the prospective subject has decided to take part in a study of his or her own volition, without coercion or any undue influence.

4. Subjects with _____ (e.g., the mentally ill or children) are vulnerable and incompetent to consent to participate in research.

5. Before a study is conducted, it must be reviewed by a committee of peers, which is called a(n) _____
    _____.

6. The three levels of institutional review of research are:

    a. _____

    b. _____

    c. _____

7. How do you assess the benefit-risk ratio of a published study? _____

    _____

    _____

    _____

    _____

    _____

    _____

    _____

    _____

    _____

    _____

    _____

8. What type of institutional review would a study probably require if it involved the review of patients' records to identify their fasting blood glucose values before surgery? _____
    _____

9. A study that involved examining the effects of a new drug on patients' serum lipid values would probably require what type of institutional review? _____.

10. Identify three different types of research misconduct.

    a. _____

    b. _____

    c. _____

11. The names of the two federal agencies that were organized for reporting and investigating research misconduct are _____ and _____ _____.

12. Is research misconduct present in nursing? Provide a rationale for your answer. _____

_____

_____

_____

_____

_____

_____

13. Are animals used in research conducted by nurses? Provide a rationale for your answer._____

_____

_____

_____

_____

_____

_____

_____

14. What agency was developed to ensure the humane treatment of animals in research? _____

_____

15. Is it appropriate to use animals as research subjects? Provide a rationale for your response. _____

_____

_____

_____

_____

_____

_____

MAKING CONNECTIONS

Historical Events, Ethical Codes, and Regulations

Directions: Match each unethical study listed below with the correct description.

a. Jewish Chronic Disease Hospital Study
b. Nazi Medical Experiments
c. Tuskegee Syphilis Study
d. Willowbrook Study

_____ 1.   Subjects were exposed to freezing temperatures, high altitudes, poisons, untested drugs, and experimental operations.

_____ 2.   The study was conducted to determine the natural course of syphilis in the adult black male.

_____ 3.   Subjects were deliberately infected with the hepatitis virus in this study.

_____ 4.   Subjects commonly were killed or sustained permanent physical, mental, or social damage during these studies.

_____ 5.   Subjects did not receive penicillin when it was identified as an effective treatment for their disease.

_____ 6.   The purpose of this study was to determine the patients' rejection responses to live cancer cells.

_____ 7.   The subjects in this study were institutionalized mentally retarded children.

_____ 8.   These experiments resulted in the development of the Nuremberg Code.

_____ 9.   The patients and physicians providing their care were unaware of the study, and it had not been approved by the IRB of the hospital.

_____ 10.   This study continued until 1972, when an account of the study appeared in the Washington Star and public outrage demanded that the study be stopped.

Ethical Principles

Directions: Match the ethical principle with the example from research.

a. Principle of beneficence
b. Principle of justice
c. Principle of respect for persons

_____ 1.   A study focused on children age 7 to 16; they were given the right to assent to participate in the study.

_____ 2.   The researcher developed a therapeutic study that would benefit the study subjects.

_____ 3.   The subjects were given the right to withdraw from the study at any time.

_____ 4.   The subjects were fairly treated by being randomly selected and assigned to a treatment or a comparison group.

_____ 5.   The subjects were promised that an interview would take only an hour of their time, and the researcher kept to a schedule of hourly interviews.

Federal Regulations Influencing the Conduct of Research

Directions: Match the federal regulation with the content or definitions provided.

a.   Department of Health and Human Services (DHHS) Protection of Human Subjects Regulations
b.   Food and Drug Administration (FDA) Protection of Human Subjects Regulations
c.   Health Insurance Portability and Accountability Act (HIPAA)

____ 1.   Regulations provide direction for conducting research with pregnant women, human fetuses, neonates, children, and prisoners.
____ 2.   Regulations were developed to protect individually identifiable health information.
____ 3.   Regulations were developed in response to the Belmont Report.
____ 4.   Regulations are focused on clinical trials to generate new drugs and refine existing drug treatments.
____ 5.   Requires that an IRB or institutional privacy board act on requests for waivers or alterations of the authorization requirement for research.

Ethics of Published Studies

Directions: Match each ethical term with the appropriate example from a published study. You can read these studies on the Elsevier website for this textbook at http://evolve.elsevier.com/burns/understanding.

a.   Coercion
b.   Diminished autonomy
c.   Fair treatment
d.   Informed consent
e.   Institutional Review Board review

Examples of Ethical Content from Published Studies

1.   Covelli (2008) conducted a study to determine the efficacy of a school-based cardiac health promotion intervention on the blood pressures of African-American adolescents. In this study, the parent/guardian signed a consent form and the participant signed an assent form, which is an example of _____.

2.   Covelli (2008, p. 175) stated "Students participated out of interest; there was no incentive for their participation." This indicates no _____ of individuals to participate in this study.

3.   Adolescents under the age of 18 have _____ to participate in research because of their age.

4.   Schultz, Goodwin, Jesseman, Toews, Lane, and Smith (2008) conducted a study to examine the effect of gel pillows on the bilateral head flattening of preterm infants. These researchers obtained consent from the hospital to conduct this study. This required what type of review? _____

5.   Schultz et al. (2008, p. 194) indicated that "Parents and legal guardians were assured that other care procedures for the infant, including repositioning, would not be altered during the study." This indicates the neonates will receive _____ during the study.

CROSSWORD PUZZLE

Directions: Complete the crossword puzzle below. Note that if the answer is more than one word, no blank spaces are left between the words.

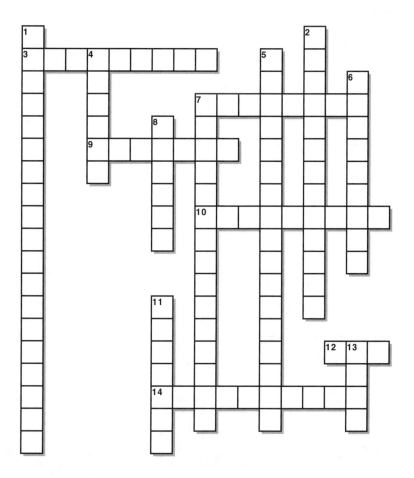

Across

3. Code developed after World War II
7. _____ are incompetent to give consent
9. Subject's permission to be in a study
10. Misinforming subjects
12. Institutional Review Board
14. Subjects who can legally choose to participate in a study or not

Down

1. Agency evaluation of a study to protect potential subjects
2. Subjects should receive _____ during a study
4. Focuses on human rights of research
5. Controlling your own fate
6. Identity of subjects unknown
7. Keeping data private
8. Child's agreement to be in a study
11. _____ act of 1974
13. Opposite of benefit, which must be examined to determine whether a study is ethical

EXERCISES IN CRITCAL APPRAISAL

Directions: Review the research articles in Appendix B to answer the following questions.

1. Is the Bindler, Massey, Shultz, Mills, and Short (2007) study ethical? Identify the information in the study that indicates that the subjects' rights were protected through informed consent, HIPAA release, and institutional review of the study.

_____

_____

_____

_____

_____

_____

_____

_____

_____

_____

_____

_____

_____

_____

_____

_____

_____

_____

2. Is the Padula, Yeaw, and Mistry (2009) study ethical? Identify the information in the study that indicates that the subjects' rights were protected through informed consent, HIPAA release, and institutional review of the study.

_____

_____

_____

_____

_____

_____

_____

_____

_____

_____

_____

_____

_____

_____

_____

_____

_____

_____

_____

3. Is the Schachman (2010) study ethical? Identify the information in the study that indicates that the subjects'
    rights were protected through informed consent, HIPAA release, and institutional review of the study.

    _____

    _____

    _____

    _____

    _____

    _____

    _____

    _____

    _____

    _____

    _____

    _____

    _____

    _____

    _____

    _____

    _____

    _____

5 Research Problems, Purposes, and Hypotheses

INTRODUCTION

You need to read Chapter 5 and then complete the following exercises. These exercises will assist you in critically appraising problems, purposes, objectives, questions, hypotheses, and variables in published studies. The answers to these exercises are in Appendix A under Chapter 5.

KEY TERMS

Directions: Match each term below with its correct definition. Each term is used only once and all terms are defined.

a. Conceptual definition of variable
b. Demographic variable
c. Dependent variable
d. Extraneous variable
e. Hypothesis
f. Independent variable

g. Operational definition of variable
h. Research problem
i. Research purpose
j. Research question
k. Research topic

Definitions

_____ 1. Variables that exist in all studies and can affect the measurement of study variables; the researcher attempts to control the influence of these variables so they do not impact the study findings.

_____ 2. Clear, concise statement of the specific goal or focus of the study that is generated from the problem.

_____ 3. Area of concern or gap in the knowledge base that is needed for practice and thus requires study.

_____ 4. Description of how variables will be measured or manipulated in a study.

_____ 5. Concise interrogative statement developed to direct a study; focuses on description of variables, examination of relationships among variables, and determination of differences between two or more groups.

_____ 6. Concept or broad problem area that provides the basis for generating numerous research problems.

_____ 7. The treatment or experimental activity that is manipulated or varied by the researcher to create an effect on the dependent variable.

_____ 8. Formal statement of the expected relationship between or expected outcome from two or more variables in a specified population.

_____ 9. Definition that provides a variable or concept with connotative (abstract, comprehensive, theoretical) meaning; established through concept analysis, concept derivation, concept synthesis, or qualitative studies.

_____ 10. The response, behavior, or outcome that is predicted or explained in research; changes in this variable are presumed to be caused by the independent variable.

_____ 11. Variables that are identified and data that are collected from the study subjects so the sample can be described.

Types of Hypotheses

Directions: Match each type of hypothesis with the correct definition.

a.   Associative hypothesis
b.   Causal hypothesis
c.   Complex hypothesis
d.   Directional hypothesis

e.   Nondirectional hypothesis
f.   Null hypothesis
g.   Research hypothesis
h.   Simple hypothesis

Definitions

_____ 1.   Hypothesis stating the relationship (associative or causal) between two variables.

_____ 2.   Alternative hypothesis to the null hypothesis; states that a relationship exists between two or more variables.

_____ 3.   Hypothesis stating a relationship between two variables in which one variable (independent variable) is thought to cause or determine the presence of the other variable (dependent variable).

_____ 4.   Hypothesis stating that a relationship exists but not predicting the exact nature of the relationship.

_____ 5.   Hypothesis predicting the relationships (associative or causal) among three or more variables.

_____ 6.   Hypothesis stating a relationship in which variables that occur or exist together in the real world are identified; thus when one variable changes, the other variables change.

_____ 7.   Hypothesis stating the specific nature of the interaction or relationship between two or more variables.

_____ 8.   Hypothesis stating that no relationships exist among the variables being studied.

Variables and Key Terms

Directions: Match each of these terms concerning variables with the appropriate example.

a.   Conceptual definition
b.   Demographic variables
c.   Dependent variables

d.   Extraneous variable
e.   Independent variable
f.   Operational definition

Definitions

_____ 1.   Pain is a physiological and psychological response to a stimulus that occurs whenever and to the degree that a patient says it does. This is an example of what type of definition?

_____ 2.   Variables that exist in all studies and can affect the measurement of study variables and affect study findings; for example, patients with fever when you are examining the effects of nasal oxygen on oral temperature. You should eliminate all patients with fever from the study because fever will affect the study's findings.

_____ 3.   The patients' pain will be measured using a visual analog scale and the Perception of Pain Likert Scale. This is an example of what type of definition?

_____ 4.   The variables of heart rate, blood pressure, and respiratory rate are measured after the completion of an exercise program.

_____ 5.   A patient receives a study intervention or treatment of ambulating every 2 hours.

_____ 6.   Variables such as age, gender, and ethnic origin are measured to describe the sample.

KEY IDEAS

Research Problem and Purpose

Directions: Fill in the blanks with the correct responses.

1. A clearly stated research purpose includes (a) _____,
    (b) _____, and usually the (c) _____
    _____.

2. Research problems and purposes are significant if they have the potential to generate and refine relevant
    knowledge that:

    a. _____

    b. _____

    c. _____

3. Identify two organizations or agencies that have developed lists of research priorities relevant to nursing.

    a. _____

    b. _____

4. The feasibility of a research problem and purpose is determined by examining the following:

    a. _____

    b. _____

    c. _____

    d. _____

5. Two ways to determine researcher expertise is by examining the _____ preparation
    and _____ experience of the researchers.

EXERCISES IN CRITICAL APPRAISAL

Bindler, Massey, Shultz, Mills, and Short (2007) Study

Directions: Review the Bindler et al. (2007) research article in Appendix B and answer the following questions.

1. State the problem of this study._____

    _____

    _____

    _____

    _____

    _____

    _____

    _____

    _____

    _____

    _____

2. State the purpose of this study. _____

    _____

    _____

    _____

    _____

    _____

    _____

    _____

3. Are the problem and the purpose significant? Provide a rationale. _____

_____

_____

_____

_____

_____

_____

_____

_____

_____

4. Does the purpose identify the variables, population, and setting for this study? _____

_____

_____

   a. Identify the variables. _____

   _____

   _____

   _____

   _____

   _____

   b. Identify the population. _____

   _____

   c. Identify the setting. _____

   _____

   _____

5. Is it feasible for the researchers to study the problem and purpose? Provide a rationale._____

_____

_____

_____

_____

_____

_____

_____

_____

_____

_____

Padula, Yeaw, and Mistry (2009) Study

Directions: Review the Padula et al. (2009) research article in Appendix B and answer the following questions.

1. State the problem of this study._____

_____

_____

_____

_____

_____

_____

_____

_____

_____

_____

2. State the purpose of this study. _____

    _____

    _____

    _____

    _____

3. Are the problem and the purpose significant? Provide a rationale. _____

    _____

    _____

    _____

    _____

    _____

    _____

    _____

    _____

4. Does the purpose identify the variables, population, and setting for this study? _____

    _____

    a. Identify the variables. _____

        _____

        _____

        _____

        _____

        _____

    b. Identify the population. _____

        _____

        _____

    c. Identify the setting. _____

        _____

        _____

5. Is it feasible for the researchers to study the problem and purpose? Provide a rationale._____

_____

_____

_____

_____

_____

_____

_____

_____

_____

_____

_____

_____

Schachman (2010) Study

Directions: Review the Schachman (2010) research article in Appendix B and answer the following questions.

1. State the problem of this study._____

_____

_____

_____

_____

_____

_____

_____

_____

_____

_____

2. State the purpose of this study. _____

   _____

   _____

   _____

   _____

   _____

3. Are the problem and the purpose significant? Provide a rationale. _____

   _____

   _____

   _____

   _____

   _____

   _____

   _____

   _____

   _____

4. Does the purpose identify the concepts or variables, population, and setting for this study? _____

   _____

   a. Identify the research concept. _____

      _____

      _____

      _____

   b. Identify the population. _____

      _____

   c. Identify the setting. _____

      _____

      _____

5. Is it feasible for the researcher to study the problem and purpose? Provide a rationale._____

_____

_____

_____

_____

_____

_____

_____

MAKING CONNECTIONS

Objectives, Questions, and Hypotheses

Directions: Ten sample hypotheses are listed below and on the next page. Identify each hypothesis using the terms listed below. Four terms are needed to identify each hypothesis. The correct answer for hypothesis #1 is provided as an example.

a. Associative hypothesis
b. Causal hypothesis
c. Complex hypothesis
d. Directional hypothesis

e. Nondirectional hypothesis
f. Null hypothesis
g. Research hypothesis
h. Simple hypothesis

<u>b, c, d, g</u> 1. Relaxation therapy is more effective than standard care in decreasing pain perception and use of pain medications in adults with chronic arthritic pain.

_____ 2. Age, family support, and health status are related to the self-care abilities of nursing home residents.

_____ 3. Heparinized saline is no more effective than normal saline in maintaining the patency and comfort of a heparin lock.

_____ 4. Poor health status is related to decreasing self-care abilities in institutionalized older adults.

_____ 5. Low-back massage is more effective in decreasing perception of low-back pain than no massage in patients with chronic low-back pain.

_____ 6. Healthy adults involved in a diet and exercise program have lower low-density lipoprotein (LDL), higher high-density lipoprotein (HDL), and lower cardiovascular risk levels than adults not involved in the program.

_____ 7. Time on the operating table, diastolic blood pressure, age, and preoperative albumin levels are related to the increased development of pressure ulcers in hospitalized older adults.

_____ 8. There are no differences in complication rates or incidence of phlebitis between patients in whom heparin locks are changed every 72 hours and those in whom locks are left in place for up to 168 hours.

_____ 9. Nurses' perceived work stress, internal locus of control, and social support are related to their psychological symptoms.

_____ 10. Cancer patients with chronic pain who listen to music with positive suggestions of pain reduction have less pain than those who do not listen to music.

11. State hypothesis #2 as a directional hypothesis. _____

_____

_____

_____

_____

_____

_____

12. State hypothesis #5 as a null hypothesis. _____

_____

_____

_____

_____

_____

_____

13. State hypothesis #9 as a null hypothesis. _____

_____

_____

_____

_____

_____

_____

EXERCISES IN CRITICAL APPRAISAL

Bindler et al. (2007) Research Article

Directions: Review the Bindler et al. (2007) research article in Appendix B and answer the following questions.

1. Are objectives, questions, or hypotheses stated in this study? Identify them._____

    _____

    _____

    _____

    _____

    _____

    _____

    _____

    _____

    _____

    _____

    _____

    _____

2. Are they appropriate and clearly stated? Provide a rationale. _____

    _____

    _____

    _____

    _____

    _____

    _____

    _____

    _____

Padula et al. (2009) Research Article

Directions: Review the Padula et al. (2009) research article in Appendix B and answer the following questions.

1   Are objectives, questions, or hypotheses stated in this study? Identify them. _____

_____

_____

_____

_____

_____

_____

_____

_____

_____

_____

_____

_____

2.   Are they appropriate and clearly stated? Provide a rationale. _____

_____

_____

_____

_____

_____

_____

_____

_____

_____

Schachman (2010) Article

Directions: Review the Schachman (2010) article in Appendix B and answer the following questions.

1. Are objectives, questions, or hypotheses stated in this study? Identify them._____

   _____

   _____

   _____

2. Are they appropriate and clearly stated? Provide a rationale. _____

   _____

   _____

   _____

MAKING CONNECTIONS

Understanding Study Variables

Directions: Match each type of variable with the sample variables provided below.

a. Demographic variable
b. Dependent variable
c. Independent variable

_____ 1.   Age
_____ 2.   Perception of pain
_____ 3.   Exercise program
_____ 4.   Gender
_____ 5.   Length of hospital stay
_____ 6.   Incidence of phlebitis
_____ 7.   Anxiety level
_____ 8.   Diet for calorie reduction

_____ 9.   Educational level
_____ 10.   Low-back massage
_____ 11.   Relaxation therapy
_____ 12.   Postoperative pain
_____ 13.   Ethnic background
_____ 14.   Total cholesterol value
_____ 15.   Marital status

EXERCISES IN CRITICAL APPRAISAL

Bindler et al. (2007) Article

Directions: Read the Bindler et al. (2007) article and answer the following questions.

1. List the major variables in this study and identify the type of each variable (independent, dependent, or research).

    Variable   **Type of Variable**

    _____

    _____

    _____

    _____

    _____

    _____

    _____

    _____

    _____

    _____

2. Identify the conceptual and operational definitions for the dependent variable: fasting serum insulin level.

    _____

    _____

    _____

    _____

    _____

    _____

    _____

    _____

    _____

    _____

3. Are these definitions clear? Provide a rationale. _____

_____

_____

_____

_____

_____

4. Identify the demographic variables in the study. _____

_____

_____

_____

_____

_____

_____

Padula et al. (2009) Article

Directions: Read the Padula et al. (2009) article and answer the following questions.

1. List the variables in this article and identify the type of each variable (independent, dependent, or research).

Variable	Type of Variable

2. Identify the conceptual and operational definitions for the independent (intervention or treatment) variable: Inspiratory Muscle Training (IMT).

    _____

    _____

    _____

    _____

    _____

    _____

    _____

    _____

    _____

3. Are these definitions clear? Provide a rationale. _____

    _____

    _____

    _____

    _____

    _____

    _____

    _____

4. Identify the demographic variables in the study. _____

    _____

    _____

    _____

    _____

    _____

Schachman (2010) Article

Directions: Read the Schachman (2010) article and answer the following questions.

1. List the major concepts or variables in this article and identify the type of each variable (independent, dependent, or research) or research concept.

   Type of Concept or Variable   **Concept or Variable**

   _____

   _____

   _____

   _____

   _____

2. Identify the conceptual definition for the research concept of the lived experience of first-time fatherhood in combat-deployed troops.

   _____

   _____

   _____

   _____

   _____

   _____

   _____

   _____

   _____

   _____

3. Is this definition clear? Provide a rationale._____

   _____

   _____

   _____

   _____

   _____

   _____

4. Identify the demographic variables in the study. _____

_____

_____

_____

_____

_____

6

Understanding the Literature Review in Published Studies

INTRODUCTION

You need to read Chapter 6 and then complete the following exercises. These exercises will assist you in reading and critically appraising research reports and summarizing the findings for use in nursing practice. The answers for the following exercises are in Appendix A under Chapter 6.

KEY TERMS

Directions: Match each term below with its correct definition. Each term is used only once and all terms are defined.

a. Academic library
b. Bibliographical database
c. Benchmarking
d. Citation
e. Complex search
f. Dissertation
g. Electronic journal
h. Evidence for best practices
i. Full-text database
j. Integrative review of research

k. Interlibrary loan department
l. Keywords
m. Link
n. Periodical
o. Primary source
p. Review of literature
q. Secondary source
r. Special library
s. Theoretical literature
t. Thesis

Definitions

_q_ 1. Source whose author summarizes or quotes content from a primary source.

_k_ 2. Department that locates books and articles in other libraries and provides the sources within a designated time.

_e_ 3. A search strategy that combines two or more keywords in one search.

_s_ 4. Literature that includes concept analyses, conceptual maps, theories, and conceptual frameworks that support a selected research problem and purpose.

_i_ 5. An electronic collection of complete journal articles.

_o_ 6. Source whose author originated or is responsible for generating the ideas published.

_r_ 7. Library that contains a collection of materials on a specific topic or specialty area, such as a library associated with a hospital.

_l_ 8. Major concepts of a topic used to begin a computer search.

_j_ 9. Review conducted to identify, analyze, and synthesize the results of independent studies to determine the current knowledge in a particular area.

_d_ 10. The author, year, title of a source, and publication information that allows a reader to find the reference to which the author is referring.

_Q_ 11. Review of theoretical and empirical sources to generate a picture of what is known and not known about a problem that provides a basis of the study conducted.

_I_ 12. A research project completed by a student as part of the requirements for a master's degree.

_B_ 13. A compilation of citations.

_C_ 14. The results of meta-analyses that are used to establish a standard of quality care.

_H_ 15. A critical appraisal and synthesis of the findings of quantitative and qualitative studies that should guide policies and procedures for patient care.

_A_ 16. Library located within an institution of higher learning that contains numerous journals and books.

_M_ 17. Moves you from one website to another website.

_F_ 18. An extensive, usually original research project that is completed by a doctoral student as part of the requirements for a doctoral degree.

_G_ 19. A journal published and available on the Internet.

_H_ 20. A literature source that is published over time and is numbered according to year.

KEY IDEAS

Directions: Fill in the blanks with the appropriate word(s).

1. The two types of sources that are reviewed and cited in a literature review for a study are _theoritical_ and _empirical_ sources.

2. The purpose of conducting a literature review in phenomenological research is to _compare & combine findings from the study_.

3. The review of literature is conducted to provide a background for the conduct of a study in _ethnographic_ and _quanitaive_ studies.

4. The literature is reviewed to develop research questions and is a source of data in _historical research_

5. Williams' (1972) study, conducted to examine factors that contribute to skin breakdown, is considered a _landmark_ study in the area of pressure ulcer prevention.

6. A literature review should include what is _known_ and _not known_ about the study problem.

7. Current sources for a literature review are defined as those that were published within _5_ years of when the article was accepted for publication.

8. Is this textbook, *Understanding Nursing Research*, an example of a primary or a secondary source? _secondary source_

9. Today, good libraries provide access to large numbers of _electronic database_ that supply a broad scope of nationally and internationally available literature.

10. Authorized users can access many library services at any time and location through the _internet_.

11. The search phase of a literature review includes the following four steps:

   a. _selecting database to search_

   b. _selecting keywords to use_

   c. _storing reference management suftware_

   d. _locating relevant literature_

12. The most frequently used database for nursing literature is _CINAHL_.

13. Most electronic databases have a(n) _thesurasus_ that can be used to identify key-word search terms.

14. Reference management software is used to _store information retrieved from computer_

15. The yearly hardbound publication, _Annual Review of Nursing Research_, is a good source for integrative reviews of research relevant to nursing practice.

16. Reviewing the literature requires a(n) _synthesis_ of the information found to determine what is known and not known about a clinical problem.

17. The written review of literature includes the following sections: _Introduction_, _empirical literature_, _theoretical literature_, and _summary_.

18. Sample research purpose: "to determine the relationship between spirituality of health care professionals and their support for family presence during invasive procedures and resuscitative efforts in adults" (Baumhover & Hughes, 2009). What keywords would you use to direct your review of literature for this study? List them in the space below.

Key terms based on the studytine to direct literature review

19. What is the difference between an integrative review of the literature and a meta-analysis?

   a. Integrative review: _Review to conduct identify, analyze & synthesize the Result from independent studies_

   b. Meta-analysis: _performing statistical analyse to ingergrate & synthesize findings completed insrvdes_

20. A search for existing literature related to a study problem requires multiple searches using various electronic databases. For each search, what should be included in a written record of the work completed?

   a. _name of database used_

   b. _date search is performed_

   c. _exact search strategy_

   d. _number of articles found_

   e. _percentage of relevant article_

MAKING CONNECTIONS

Theoretical and Empirical Sources

Directions: Theoretical and empirical writings are included in the literature review of a published study. Read the sources below and label each with a T if it is a theoretical source or an E if it is an empirical source. The final determination of the type of source would be made by reviewing the source.

T 1.   Lazarus, R. S., & Folkman, S. (1984). *Stress, appraisal, and coping.* New York: Springer.

E 2.   Abstracts from a research conference

E 3.   Master's thesis

T 4.   Jackson, J. R., Clements, P. T., Averill, J. B., & Zimbro, K. (2009). Patterns of knowing: Proposing a theory for nursing leadership. *Nursing Economic$, 27*(3), 149-159.

T 5.   Orem, D. E., Taylor, S., & Renpenning, K. M. (2001). *Nursing: Concepts of practice* (6th ed.) St. Louis: Mosby.

E 6.   Sammarco, A., & Konecny, L. M. (2010). Quality of life, social support, and uncertainty among Latina and Caucasian breast cancer survivors: A comparative study. *Oncology Nursing Forum, 37*(1), 93-99.

E 7.   Smith, R., & Porock, D. (2009). Caring for people dying at home: A research study into the needs of community nurses. *International Journal of Palliative Nursing, 15*(12), 601-608.

E 8.   Doctoral dissertation

T 9.   von Bertalanffy, L. (1968). *General systems theory.* New York: Braziller.

T 10. Lewin's Change Theory

E 11. Jones, R. A. (2010). Patient education in rural community hospitals: Registered nurses' attitudes and degrees of comfort. *Journal of Continuing Education in Nursing, 41*(1), 41-48.

T 12. Kübler-Ross, E. (1969). *On death and dying.* New York: Macmillan.

Primary and Secondary Sources

Directions: A literature review includes mainly primary sources. Remember that a primary source is developed by the person conducting the research or developing the theory. A secondary source is the synthesis of primary and other sources. Based on these definitions, determine if a source is primary or secondary. Label each source below with a P if it is a primary source or an S if it is a secondary source.

S 1.   Integrated review of research

P 2.   Doctoral dissertation

P 3.   Master's thesis

S 4.   Textbook

S 5.   Summary of theoretical and empirical sources

P 6.   Study published in *Applied Nursing Research*

P 7.   Landmark study of pressure ulcers

S 8.   Published review of literature article

P 9.   Exact replication of a study

P 10. Historical research article in *Image: Journal of Nursing Scholarship*

The Purpose of the Literature Review in Quantitative Research Methodologies

In a quantitative research report, the literature that is cited can be for what purposes? List four ways literature is used in a quantitative report.

a. Summeraize background

b. describe theoretical framework

c. Justify methods of study

d. Compare Results

The Literature in Qualitative Research Methods

Directions: Each different research method in qualitative research uses the literature in a slightly different way. Match the qualitative research method below with the phrase that describes how researchers using that method primarily use the literature.

Qualitative Research Methods

a. Phenomenological research
b. Grounded theory research
c. Ethnographical research
d. Historical research

How the Method Primarily Uses the Literature

D 1. Is the source of data
C 2. Provides background for the study
A 3. Compares and combines findings
B 4. Supports the findings or theory developed

Critically Appraising the Literature Review

List five questions that should be considered when critically appraising a literature review section of a published study.

a. identify primary & secondary sources

b. Are studies current

c. Review organized

d. Review logical

e. Studies pharaphrase

Performing Literature Searches

Match the type of library to the publications listed below. You will use the types of libraries more than once and some publications are in more than one library so they will have more than one answer.

a. Academic library at a liberal arts university
b. Public library
c. Special library at a school of medicine
d. Special library at an alternative treatment center

C 1. Unpublished papers of a deceased medical researcher
B 2. Children's book for hospitalized child
A,C 3. Bound periodical from 2005
B 4. Best-selling fiction paperback
A 5. Textbooks on sociology
D 6. Patient teaching materials on acupuncture
A,C 7. This month's issue of a peer-reviewed radiology journal
A 8. Book on a theory of psychosocial environment
A,C 9. *Journal of the American Medical Association*
A 10. *Journal of Nursing Scholarship*

11. What word is used in complex literature searches to combine keywords? AND

12. List four different electronic databases commonly searched by nurses.

   a. CINAHL
   b. OVID
   c. EBSCO
   d. MEDLINE

Writing a Review of Literature

In the space below, describe the sections and their purposes in a written review of literature.

   a. Introduction
   b. Critical Apraisial
   c. Conceptual framework
   d. The summary

CROSSWORD PUZZLE

Directions: Complete the crossword puzzle below. Note: If the answer is more than one word, no blank spaces are left between the words.

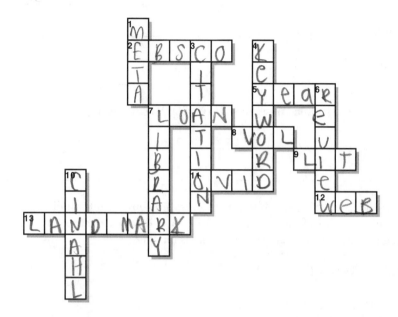

Across

2. Electronic bibliographic database
5. 365 days
7. Interlibrary _____
8. Shortened word for "volume"
9. Shortened word for "literature"
11. Electronic full-text database
12. Internet
13. Classic study

Down

1. _____-analysis
3. Author, year, title, journal, volume, pages
4. Major concept in a search
6. Summary
7. Place that contains books and journals
10. Abbreviation for Cumulative Index to Nursing & Allied Health Literature

EXERCISES IN CRITICAL APPRAISAL

Directions: Review the following three articles in Appendix B: Bindler et al. (2007), Padula et al. (2009), and Schachman (2010). Use these articles to answer the following questions.

1. The most common way to cite a reference is the American Psychological Association (APA) (2009) format. Knowing the different parts of a reference citation will assist you in locating and recording sources for a formal paper. The following source is presented in APA format. Please write the category of the citation information in the spaces provided.

   Schachman, K. A. (2010). Online fathering: The experience of first-time fatherhood in combat-deployed troops. *Nursing Research, 59*(1), 11-17.

   a. In this reference, *Nursing Research* is the _____.

   b. In this reference, the 2010 is _____.

   c. In this reference, the 59 is _____.

   d. In this reference, the 11-17 refers to the _____.

   e. In this reference, the 1 represents the _____.

   f. Who is the author of this article? _____.

   g. What is the title of the article? _____
   _____

2. Write the reference for the Padula, Yeaw, and Mistry (2009) article using APA (2009) format._____

_____

_____

3. Incomplete and incorrect references in published studies are a problem for individuals trying to locate sources from the reference list of the article. The following reference citations from the Schachman (2010) article are missing at least one element. Indicate what is missing.

   a. Draper, J. (2003). *Nursing Inquiry, 10*(1).

      What is missing? _____

   b. Premberg, A., Hellstrom, A. L., & Berg, M. (2008). Experiences of the first year as father. *Scandinavian Journal of Caring Sciences*, (1)

      What is missing? _____

   c. Barclay, L., & Lupton, D. The experiences of new fatherhood: A socio-cultural analysis. *Journal of Advanced Nursing*, 1013-1020.

      What is missing? _____

   _____

4. What are the titles for the sections of the following articles that include the studies' literature review?

   a. Padula, Yeaw, & Mistry (2009): _____

   b. Bindler, Massey, Shultz, Mills, & Short (2007): _____

5. In the article written by Schachman (2010) about her qualitative study, in which sections did she incorporate the review of the literature?

_____

_____

_____

6. Are relevant studies identified and described in the Padula et al. (2009) literature review? Give examples of two studies that are cited in the literature review of the article.

_____

_____

_____

_____

_____

_____

_____

7. Are relevant theoretical explanations identified and described in the review of the literature of the Padula et al. (2009) study?

_____

_____

_____

_____

_____

_____

8. What type of source was used to support the nursing intervention, an empirical or a theoretical source?

_____

9. In Padula et al. (2009) study references, is the source by Caroci and Lareau (2004) a primary or a secondary source? _____

10. Are the references in the Padula et al. (2009) study current? Provide a rationale._____

_____

_____

_____

_____

_____

_____

_____

11. Does the literature review in the Padula et al. (2009) study present the current knowledge base for the research problem? How would you determine this? Provide a rationale for your answer.

_____

_____

_____

_____

_____

_____

_____

_____

12. Are relevant studies identified and described in the Bindler et al. (2007) study? Provide two examples.

_____

_____

_____

_____

_____

_____

_____

13. Are relevant theories identified and described in the Bindler et al. (1997) study? Identify one theoretical source that is cited in the study's literature review.

_____

_____

_____

_____

_____

_____

_____

14. In the Bindler et al. (2007) study references, is the source by Steinberger and Daniels (2003) a primary or a secondary source? _____

    Is the source by Weigensberg et al. (2005) a primary or a secondary source? _____

15. Are the references in the Bindler et al. (2007) study current? Provide a rationale. _____

    _____

    _____

    _____

    _____

    _____

    _____

16. Does the literature review in the Bindler et al. (2007) study provide a current knowledge base for the research problem examined in this study? Provide a rationale.

    _____

    _____

    _____

    _____

    _____

    _____

    _____

    _____

17. Are relevant studies identified and described in the Schachman (2010) study? Give examples of two studies that are cited in the literature review of the article.

    _____

    _____

    _____

    _____

    _____

    _____

    _____

18. Are relevant theories identified and described in the Schachman (2010) study? Identify one theoretical source that is cited in the study's literature review.

_____

_____

_____

19. In Schachman's (2010) references, is the book by Hodnett et al. (2007) a primary or a secondary source?
_____

Is the source by Premberg et al. (2008) a primary or a secondary source? _____

20. Are the references in Schachman's (2010) study current? Provide a rationale._____

_____

_____

_____

_____

_____

_____

_____

21. Does the literature review of Schachman's (2010) study provide the current knowledge base of the problem examined in this study? Provide a rationale.

_____

_____

_____

_____

Reference

Baumhover, N., & Hughes, L. (2009). Spirituality and support for family presence during invasive procedures and resuscitation efforts in adults. *American Journal of Critical Care, 18*(4), 357-367.

7 Understanding Theory and Research Frameworks

INTRODUCTION

You need to read Chapter 7 and then complete the following exercises. These exercises will assist you in learning key terms and identifying and critically appraising frameworks in published studies. The answers for the following exercises are in Appendix A under Chapter 7.

KEY TERMS

Directions: Match each term below with its correct definition. Each term is used only once and all terms are defined.

a. Abstract thinking
b. Assumption
c. Concept
d. Conceptual map for a study
e. Conceptual model
f. Construct

g. Framework
h. Middle-range theory
i. Proposition
j. Scientific theory
k. Theory

Definitions

_____ 1. An abstract, logical structure of meaning that guides the development of a study, is often tested in the study, and enables the researcher to link the findings to nursing's body of knowledge.

_____ 2. Includes abstract constructs that explain a phenomenon, express assumptions, and reflect a philosophical stance. Orem developed one of these to describe professional nursing.

_____ 3. Thinking oriented toward the development of a general idea, without association with a particular instance.

_____ 4. Diagram showing the interrelationship between concepts presented in a study.

_____ 5. Statements that are considered true without testing.

_____ 6. A type of theory that has been extensively tested through research and includes clear definitions of concepts and factual relationships.

_____ 7. Organized set of concepts and statements that serve to describe, explain, and predict an event or phenomenon.

_____ 8. A term that abstractly names an object or phenomenon.

_____ 9. A type of theory that is commonly used as a framework in research.

_____ 10. Highly abstract ideas used in constructing conceptual models.

_____ 11. Abstract statement describing a relationship among concepts that make up a middle-range theory and usually one or two are tested in a study.

KEY IDEAS

Directions: Fill in the blanks in this section with the appropriate word(s) or number(s).

1. We use theories to _____.

2. Testing a theory involves _____.

3. _____ are not generally considered testable in research.

4. Research needs to be based on theory that is present in a study as a(n) _____.

5. A framework that has been used rather shallowly to provide an overall orientation for a study but does not guide the study is referred to as _____.

6. Research findings are interpreted in terms of _____.

7. In a framework, all _____ should be defined.

8. Terms or ideas in conceptual models are referred to as _____.

9. A(n) _____ is more specific than a concept and is defined so that it is measurable in a study.

10. The _____ of a theory are tested through research.

11. Statements at the lowest level of abstraction presented in a study are referred to as _____ _____.

12. The purpose of a conceptual map is to _____.

13. A conceptual map includes _____.

14. An organized program of research designed to build a body of knowledge related to a particular conceptual model is referred to as a(n) _____.

15. Another term for a practice theory is _____ theory.

16. Which is more specific? (Choose one): Variable or Concept

17. The five essential elements of a framework used in a study include:

    a. _____

    b. _____

    c. _____

    d. _____

    e. _____

18. _____ a framework involves identification and evaluation of concepts, definitions, and propositions of the theory tested in the study.

19. When a study's framework is not clearly identified, it is called a(n) _____ framework.

20. List five middle-range theories:

    a. _____

    b. _____

    c. _____

    d. _____

    e. _____

21. Pender has a middle-range theory about _____.

22. The theorist named _____ has a model of self-care.

MAKING CONNECTIONS

Levels of Abstraction

Directions: Place the following terms in order from the highest to the lowest level of abstraction.

Variable   **Construct**   **Operational definition**   **Concept**

[Highest level of abstraction]

_____

_____

_____

_____

[Lowest level of abstraction]

Elements of Theory

Directions: Study the diagram below and answer the following questions in the spaces provided.

Physical Health ———— + ⟶ Quality of Life

Psychological Health ⟶ +

1. List the concepts in the diagram. _____

    _____

    _____

2. What do the arrows represent? _____

_____

_____

_____

3. What does this figure represent when included in a study? _____

_____

_____

Examples of Frameworks

Directions: Several theories were identified in Chapter 7 that had been used in studies. Match the name of the theory to the appropriate theorist's name. Hint—Review the middle-range theories in Table 7-5.

Theory

____ 1. Self-Efficacy

____ 2. Acute Pain

____ 3. Health Belief Model

____ 4. Dyspnea

____ 5. Stress, Appraisal, and Coping

____ 6. Resilience

____ 7. Planned Behavior

____ 8. Uncertainty in Illness

Theorist

a. Polk, 1997

b. Mischel, 1988

c. Gift, 1992

d. Ajzen, 1991

e. Lazarus and Folkman, 1984

f. Bandura, 1986

g. Becker, 1976

h. Good, 1998

CROSSWORD PUZZLE

Directions: Complete the crossword puzzle below. Note: If the answer is more than one word, no blank spaces are left between the words.

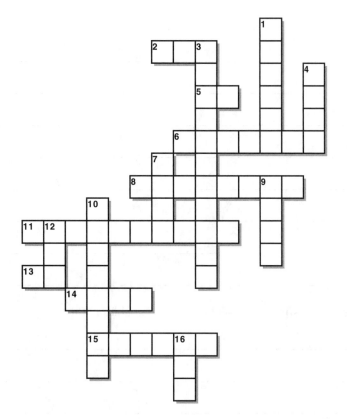

Across

2. Conceptual diagram
5. Either/_____
6. The basic element of a theory
8. Measured in a study
11. Testable prediction in a study
13. A, E, I, __, __
14. Self-deficit theory
15. Integrated set of concepts and statements

Down

1. _____-range theory
3. Relational statement
4. Examination
7. Self-_____
9. Represented by an arrow
10. Opposite of abstract
12. Us = me and _____
16. Adaptation theorist

EXERCISES IN CRITICAL APPRAISAL

Directions: Examine the framework of Bindler, Massey, Shultz, Mills, and Short (2007) study provided in Appendix B.

1. List the concepts in the study. Hint—There are four major concepts in this study. _____

_____

_____

_____

_____

2. State the definition of each concept as defined by the author(s). Are the definitions clear and adequate? If not, identify the inadequacies.

_____

_____

_____

_____

_____

_____

_____

_____

_____

3. List the variables used in the study. Hint—There are 13 variables in this study._____

_____

_____

_____

_____

_____

_____

_____

_____

_____

4.   Link the concepts below with the appropriate study variable.

Concept	Variable(s)
Metabolic syndrome	
Lifestyle and environment	
Genetics	

5.   Complete the following table by listing each concept, the related variable(s), and the measurement method(s).

Concept	Variable(s)	Measurement Method(s)
Metabolic syndrome		
Lifestyle and environment		
Genetics		

6. Does the Bindler et al. (2007) study have a clearly identified framework? What theory do you think provides a basis for this study?

_____

_____

_____

_____

_____

_____

_____

Directions: Examine the framework of Padula, Yeaw, and Mistry (2009) study provided in Appendix B.

1. Does Padula et al. (2009) have a clearly identified framework? If so, what is the name of the theorist and theory that provided the framework for this study?

_____

_____

_____

2. List the major concepts that were the focus of this study. Hint—There are six major concepts in this study that are linked to study variables.

_____

_____

_____

_____

_____

3. State the definition of the concept self-efficacy as defined by the authors._____

_____

_____

_____

_____

4. List the one independent variable and five dependent variables examined in this study. _____

_____

_____

_____

_____

5. Link the following concepts with the variables in the Padula et al. (2009) study.

Concept	Variable(s)
Situational demands	
Vicarious experiences Verbal persuasion Enactive attainment	
Performance accomplishment Enhanced self-efficacy	

6. Complete the following table by listing each concept, the related variable(s), and the measurement method(s) for dependent variables and manipulation of independent variable.

Concept	Variable(s)	Measurement Method(s) for Dependent Variables and Manipulation of Independent Variable
Situational demands		
Vicarious experiences Verbal persuasion Enactive attainment		
Performance accomplishment Enhanced self-efficacy		

7. Does Padula et al. (2009) provide a model or map of their study framework? _____

_____

_____

Nicole Nelson, BSN, RN, a master's in nursing student at the University of Texas at Arlington, developed the following map and description for the Padula et al. (2009) study.

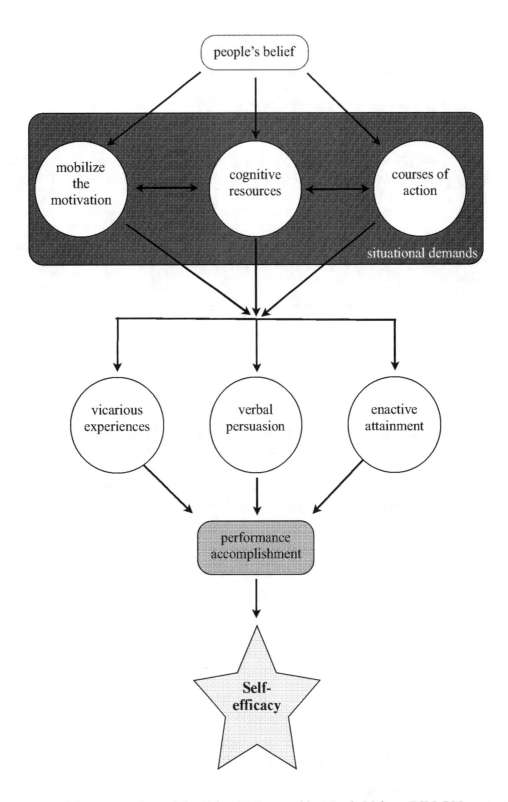

Figure 7-1. Map and description for Padula et al. (2009) created by Nicole Nelson, BSN, RN.

This model or map displays the self-efficacy process. In my opinion, a person's belief is at the beginning of the self-efficacy process because their background and belief system form a foundation to how they will perform in a particular manner to attain certain goals. All of the shapes in the model, except for the star, are in a circular form to display the continuation of each concept. The arrows directing downward from people's belief display a positive directional causal relationship to mobilize the motivation, cognitive resources and courses of action. All three of these concepts are dependent on the person to utilize their own capabilities. People need to be able to motivate themselves, have people around them for cognitive and mental support, and the ability to have courses of action in place to obtain their goals. Surrounding these concepts is the larger figure of situational demands, because external and internal factors can easily change a person and their goal setting. From each of the three concepts located within situational demands is a positive directional causal relationship down to a common line that links the relationship to each of the interventions of goal achievement.

The concepts of vicarious experiences, verbal persuasion, and enactive attainment are each located within a circle to display the influence of these concepts in affecting a person on their path to self-efficacy. From these three concepts, a positive directional causal relationship exists to enable performance accomplishment. The positive directional causal relationship continues further to the goal of enhanced self-efficacy. The star was chosen because in my opinion it symbolizes the final step in the achievement of a person's goals. Each of the relationships in this model are positive, directional, and causal; because if a person believes they can obtain an objective, then they will mobilize their motivation to gain what they are seeking and if a person is able to formulate a course of action then they can use their vicarious experiences to help them obtain the ultimate goal of enhanced self-efficacy (Nelson, 2010).

8 Clarifying Quantitative Research Designs

INTRODUCTION

You need to read Chapter 8 and then complete the following exercises. These exercises will assist you in learning key terms and identifying and critically appraising designs in published studies. The answers for these exercises are in Appendix A under Chapter 8.

KEY TERMS

Directions: Match each term below with its correct definition. Each term is used only once and all terms are defined.

a. Bias
b. Causality
c. Control
d. Correlational design
e. Dependent variable
f. Descriptive design
g. Design

h. Independent variable
i. Manipulation
j. Multicausality
k. Pretest
l. Probability
m. Randomized clinical trial
n. Replication study

Definitions

A 1. Distortion of study findings or to deviate from the true or expected.

G 2. Blueprint for conducting a study.

B 3. Particular cause leads to specific effect(s) or outcome(s).

L 4. Addresses relative rather than absolute causality.

D 5. To examine relationships between or among two or more variables in a single group.

C 6. The power to direct or manipulate factors to achieve a desired outcome. This is greater in experimental than quasi-experimental designs.

K 7. Obtaining baseline information or data from a sample.

J 8. The recognition that several interrelating variables can be involved in causing a particular effect.

F 9. Study design to gain more information about characteristics in a particular field of study.

N 10. Study is repeated to verify initial results.

i 11. Controlling a treatment or intervention in an experimental study.

e 12. Effect or outcome variable.

h 13. Cause or experimental variable.

m 14. Complex study investigating effects of treatments such as drugs.

KEY IDEAS

Directions: Fill in the blanks in this section with the appropriate word(s) or number(s).

1. According to causality theory, things have causes and causes lead to _effects_.

2. From the perspective of probability, a(n) _cause_ may not produce a specific _effect_ each time that particular _cause_ occurs.

3. Designs are developed to reduce the possibilities and effects of _biases_.

4. The purpose of quasi-experimental and experimental research designs is to maximize _control_ of factors in the study situation.

5. The focus of a quasi-experimental study is the manipulation of _treatment_.

6. Critical appraisal of research involves being able to think through threats to _design validity_ that have occurred and make judgments about how seriously they affect the integrity of the findings.

7. Quasi-experimental and experimental studies are designed to examine _cause & effect_.

8. When a phenomenon is caused by many factors, this is called _multicausality_.

9. A study critical appraisal should look for possible sources of _bias_.

10. A researcher wants to _control_ the design of a study by limiting it only to first-time elderly (>40 years) mothers.

11. The study design that has the highest level of control is a(n) _experimental design_.

12. Control is usually limited in _correlational studies_ studies.

13. The _comparative descrip._ design is used to examine descriptively the differences between two groups, such as the difference between males and females for surgical anxiety.

14. _correlational_ studies are conducted to examine relationships among variables.

15. Model testing designs may be used to test _middle range theories_.

16. The least _error_ with the most control is seen in experimental research designs.

17. List three elements of experimental designs:

    a. _Control of setting_

    b. _Random factor_

    c. _Comparison group_

18. A quasi-experimental design has less _control_ than experimental designs.

19. Randomized clinical trials should have large or small sample sizes? _large_

20. List three different types of interventions.

a. Social

b. educational

c. environmental

MAKING CONNECTIONS

Control and Designs for Nursing Studies

Directions: For each of the questions below, identify the most appropriate research design or study and provide a rationale for your answers. What elements might be controlled, if any? Each type of design or study is used only once.

Choices:

✓Case study design   ✓Comparative descriptive design   ✓Descriptive study
✓Experimental design   Model testing design   ✓Quasi-experimental design—
✓Quasi-experimental design   ✓Replication study   two posttests
✓Survey design   ✓Randomized clinical trial

1. Effectiveness of a new drug to treat hypertension in adults. The study had a large sample of convenience and included all patients with hypertension in five primary care clinics. Subjects were randomly assigned to either the treatment or comparison groups.

     Randomized clinical trial - test new drug, have
     diff. doses races, & ages

2. Determining the effectiveness of a patient pain-scoring system in 5-year-old children. The study had experimental and comparison groups and a sample size of 80, with 40 children in each group. The subjects were obtained by a sample of convenience, with 40 children from one hospital unit and 40 from another unit.

     Quasi-experimental - effect of new pain scale
     vs the old pain scale

3. In-depth description of a nursing school's class of 2011. *Case Study –*
    To Study the new nursing class

4. Survey of nurses' attitudes regarding at-home hemodialysis. *Descriptive study –*
    identify, describe home health ~~patient~~ care &
    their experiences

5. Conducting a master's thesis that repeats a previous study. *~~Descriptive study~~*
    Replication study – determine similar patterns

6. Identifying and describing the health-promotion behaviors of patients experiencing their first myocardial infarction (MI).
    Descriptive Study – identify & describe home
    health promotion tips

7. Describing and examining the differences in health-promotion behaviors for males and females with diabetes.

    Comparative - describe differences to male & female

8. Examining the effect of vitamins on weight gain in children who have failure to thrive at 6 months and 1 year. The experimental group is selected from one primary care office and the comparison group from another primary care office.

    Quasi Experimental 2 posttest - examing the results of vitamins in wergnt gain at 6 months & also a year

9. Testing the Orem self-care model to predict the self-care behaviors in diabetic adolescents. _____

    Model - Testing Design - To predict self help behaviors in teens (diabetic)

10. Randomly select women with lung cancer and randomly assign them to treatment or nontreatment groups to determine the effectiveness of a new chemotherapy agent on tumor size. Extensive control of treatment, measurement of tumor size, and data collection process.

    Experimental Study Design - new chemomerapy on me size of the tumor

Mapping the Design

Directions: Map the following designs in the space below each type of design. Refer to your textbook to help you with the different types of designs.

259 1. Typical descriptive design with four study variables: *describe selected variables*

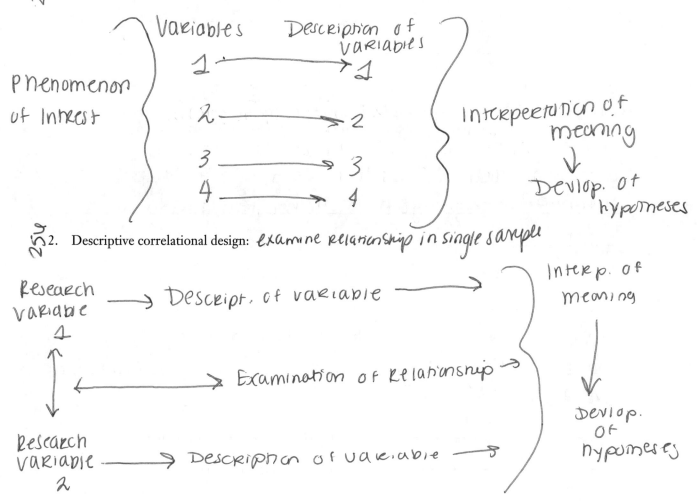

25u 2. Descriptive correlational design: *examine relationship in single sample*

275 3. Quasi-experimental pretest and posttest design with comparison group: *convience & random assignment*

CROSSWORD PUZZLE

Directions: Complete the crossword puzzle below. Note: If the answer is more than one word, no blank spaces are left between the words.

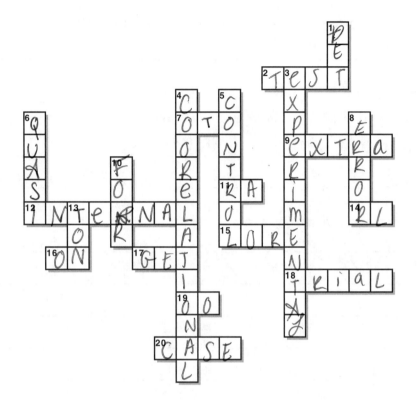

Across

2. Post-
7. Map in studies for experimental group
9. One more than needed
11. Egyptian sun god
12. Design validity within conduct of study
14. Abbreviation for "right/left"
15. Folk story
16. Place it _____ the table
17. To obtain
18. Randomized clinical _____
19. Map in experimental studies for control group
20. Single unit study

Down

1. Animal friend
3. Design with precise control
4. Design of variable relationships
5. Researcher has power or _____ over design
6. _____-experimental design
8. Mistake
10. _____ and function
13. 2000 pounds

EXERCISES IN CRITCAL APPRAISAL

Directions: Examine the design of Bindler, Massey, Shultz, Mills, and Short (2007) study in Appendix B, and answer the following questions.

1. Identify the type of design used in this study. <u>Predictive correlational design</u>

2. What comparisons were made in the Bindler et al. (2007) study? <u>The 3 ethinic groups:</u> <u>Native Americans, Hispanic, Causain. Also their</u> <u>demographic group, physical MET score, biophysiologic cholesterol measures.</u>

3. Identify three strengths in the design.

   a. <u>Data was collected on time in the same setting</u>

   b. <u>Subjects were all from different races</u>

   c. <u>They use an expert for their expernise (dietitan)</u>

4. Identify three sources of potential bias in this study.

   a. <u>Used a recall method of for measuring</u>

   b. <u>People volunteered wasn't Random</u>

   c. <u>All ethnic groups didn't have the same number</u>

5. List three methods of control used in the Bindler et al. (2007) design.

   a. <u>Controlling measurement: BP taken 3 times & they used average</u>

   b. <u>Control over environment: All used same setting</u>

   c. <u>Control of extroneous variables: took blood properly</u>

6. To what population(s) can the findings be generalized? Provide a rationale. _____

Different ethnic groups of people in the 4th–8th grade who lived in a rural area. Hispanics had the greatest number of participants.

Directions: Examine the design of the Padula, Yeaw, and Mistry (2009) study found in Appendix B, and answer the following questions.

1. Identify the type of design used in this study. _Quasi Experimental Design_

2. What comparisons were made in the Padula et al. (2009) study? _effects of treatment made for both the control & experimental group of healthcare_

3. Identify three strengths in the Padula et al. (2009) study design.

   a. _Random assignment → Coin toss_
   b. _Detailed plan for eliminating Risk_
   c. _Followed sample criteria_

4. Identify three sources of potential bias in the Padula et al. (2009) study.

   a. _Orginial sample wasn't Random_
   b. _Small sample size_
   c. _~~scribbled~~ pt. Journals_

5. List three methods of control used in the Padula et al. (2009) study design.

    a. _extensive Control to comply_

    b. _measurement of physiologic factors_

    c. _ethical aspect_

6. To what population(s) can the findings be generalized? Provide a rationale. _____

    The IMT & it's effectiveness for parents w/ HF.

    Heelped pt. but not ᵈⁱᵃⁿᵗ determine pt.'s self-efficacy.

9 Examining Populations and Samples in Research

INTRODUCTION

You need to read Chapter 9 and then complete the following exercises. These exercises will assist you in understanding and critically appraising the sampling process in published studies. The answers to these exercises are in Appendix A under Chapter 9.

KEY TERMS

Directions: Match each term below with its correct definition. Each term is used only once and all terms are defined.

a. Accessible population
b. Cluster sampling
c. Convenience sampling
d. Network sampling
e. Nonprobability sampling
f. Probability sampling
g. Purposive sampling
h. Quota sampling

i. Simple random sampling
j. Sampling
k. Sampling criteria
l. Stratified random sampling
m. Systematic sampling
n. Target population
o. Theoretical sampling

Definitions

_____ 1. Process of selecting a group of people, events, behaviors, or other elements that are representative of the population being studied.

_____ 2. Portion of the target population to which the researcher has reasonable access.

_____ 3. All elements (individuals, objects, events, or substances) that meet the sampling criteria for inclusion in a study.

_____ 4. Judgmental sampling that involves the conscious selection by the researcher of certain subjects or elements to include in a study.

_____ 5. List of the characteristics essential for membership in the target population.

_____ 6. Random sampling technique in which every member (element) of the population has a probability higher than zero of being selected for the sample; examples include simple random sampling, stratified random sampling, cluster sampling, and systematic sampling.

_____ 7. Sampling technique selecting every *k*th individual from an ordered list of all members of a population, using a randomly selected starting point.

_____ 8. Random selection of subjects from the sampling frame for a study.

_____ 9. Random sampling technique used when the researcher knows some of the variables in the population that are critical to achieving representativeness; the sample is divided into strata or groups using these identified variables.

____ 10. Sampling technique in which a frame is developed that includes a list of all states, cities, institutions, or organizations that could be used in a study; a randomized sample is drawn from this list.

____ 11. Snowballing technique that takes advantage of social networks and the fact that friends tend to hold characteristics in common; subjects meeting sample criteria are asked to assist in locating others with similar characteristics.

____ 12. Sampling in which not every element of the population has an opportunity for selection, such as convenience sampling, quota sampling, purposive sampling, and network sampling.

____ 13. Convenience sampling technique with an added strategy to ensure the inclusion of subjects who are likely to be underrepresented in the convenience sample, such as women and minority groups.

____ 14. Sampling technique that involves including subjects in a study because they happened to be in the right place at the right time.

____ 15. A sampling method often used in grounded theory research to develop a selected theory through the research process.

KEY IDEAS

Directions: Fill in the blanks with the appropriate word(s).

1. The individual units of a population are called _____.

2. The sample is obtained from the accessible population and is generalized to the _____
_____.

3. Representativeness means that the _____, _____
_____, and _____
_____ are alike in as many ways as possible.

4. Identify two ways you might evaluate the representativeness of a sample in a published study.

   a. _____

   b. _____

5. Random variation is_____
_____.

6. A list of every member of a population is referred to as a(n) _____.

7. A sampling plan outlines the _____
_____.

8. In critically appraising the sampling plan in a study, what three things might you examine?

   a. _____

   b. _____

   c. _____

9. When the sampling criteria are narrowly defined or very specific, the sample desired is more _____
_____.

10. When the sampling criteria are broadly defined to include a variety of subjects, the sample desired is more _____.

11. Subjects must be over the age of 18, able to read and write English, newly diagnosed with cancer, and have no other major illnesses. These are examples of _____.

12. The sample was 65% female and 40% African American, 30% Hispanic, and 30% Caucasian, which are examples of _____.

13. When subjects are lost to a study, it is referred to as _____.

14. The use of the term *control group* is limited to those studies using _____ sampling methods.

15. If _____ sampling methods are used for sample selection, the group not receiving the treatment is referred to as a *comparison group*.

16 Identify four types of probability sampling.

    a. _____

    b. _____

    c. _____

    d. _____

17. When subjects are randomly selected and then randomly assigned to treatment or control groups, this is a _____ sampling technique.

18. Identify four types of nonprobability sampling.

    a. _____

    b. _____

    c. _____

    d. _____

19. Currently, do the majority of nursing studies use probability or nonprobability sampling methods? _____

20. Convenience sampling is also called _____.

21. Purposive sampling is referred to as _____.

22. The adequacy of the sample size in quantitative studies can be evaluated using _____ _____.

23. Power is the capacity to detect _____ or _____ that actually exist in the population.

24. The minimal acceptable level of power for a study is _____.

25. If the findings of a study are nonsignificant, the researcher should examine the adequacy of the sample size by running a(n) _____.

26. Effect size is the extent to which the _____ is false.

27. Identify five factors that influence the adequacy of a study's sample size in quantitative studies.

    a. _____

    b. _____

    c. _____

    d. _____

    e. _____

28. Identify the types of research settings used in nursing studies.

    a. _____

    b. _____

    c. _____

29. The two types of sampling criteria that might be used in a study are _____ and _____ criteria.

30. Calculate the refusal rate for a study in which 250 potential subjects were approached, 217 accepted participation, and 33 refused participation. What percent of the potential subjects refused to participate?

    _____

MAKING CONNECTIONS

Sampling Methods for Quantitative and Qualitative Studies

Directions: Match the appropriate sampling method with the example sampling information from a study. Some of the sampling methods might be used more than once.

a. Cluster sampling
b. Convenience sampling
c. Network sampling
d. Purposive sampling
e. Quota sampling

f. Simple random sampling
g. Stratified random sampling
h. Systematic sampling
i. Theoretical sampling

_____ 1. A sample of 500 nurses was randomly selected from a list of all registered nurses in the state of Texas.

_____ 2. A sample of 50 diabetic patients was obtained from an outpatient clinic and randomly placed in the comparison and experimental groups.

_____ 3. A sample of 10 subjects with HIV was obtained by asking three subjects to identify friends with HIV who might participate in the study.

_____ 4. A sample of 1000 critical care nurses was obtained by asking 100 critical care nurse managers in 50 randomly selected, large hospitals to identify 10 staff nurses to complete a survey.

_____ 5. A sample of 50 subjects was asked to participate in a study at an immunization booth in the mall.

_____ 6. Gender was used to stratify a sample of 100 randomly selected subjects.

_____ 7. The researcher obtained a list of all certified nurse practitioners, picked a random starting point, and then selected every 25th individual to participate in the study.

_____ 8. A sample of 50 hypertensive subjects was recruited in a clinic to participate in a study.

_____ 9. An equal number of patients with asthma, emphysema, and chronic bronchitis were recruited from the local Better Breathers Chapter and asked to participate in a study.

_____ 10. The sample included 50 patients; 25 were examples of strong self-care and 25 were examples of poor self-care.

_____ 11. A sample of 5000 military personnel was randomly selected to participate in a study.

_____ 12. A sample of 10 drug-addicted nurses was obtained by asking five subjects to identify friends who were drug addicted.

_____ 13. A sample of 15 home health patients was asked to participate in a study because they had what were determined to be stage IV pressure ulcers that were not healing.

_____ 14. A sample of 50 adolescents was obtained at a fast-food restaurant.

_____ 15. A sample of 50 surgery patients was randomly selected from a hospital and randomly placed in control and treatment groups.

_____ 16. Starting from a random point, every 10th subject who entered the emergency department was selected for participation in the study until a sample of 100 was achieved.

_____ 17. A grounded theory study was conducted to develop a theory about response to hurricane disaster, and a sample was selected to promote generation of the theory.

_____ 18. A sample of 80 heart transplant patients was obtained by asking 20 critical care nurse managers in 20 randomly selected, large urban hospitals to identify 4 patients to participate in a study.

_____ 19. A sample of 10 subjects who had experienced sexual assault was selected; 5 of them were considered to be coping well after the assault, and 5 were considered to be coping very poorly after the assault. Data saturation was achieved with these 10 subjects.

_____ 20. A sample of 150 subjects receiving care in a university health center was asked to participate in a study.

Determining Sample Size for Quantitative and Qualitative Research

Directions: Match the type of research, quantitative or qualitative, with the criteria for determining the appropriate sample size for a study.

a. Qualitative research

b. Quantitative research

c. Both qualitative and quantitative research

_____ 1. Sample size is adequate when saturation of information is achieved in the study area.

_____ 2. The scope of the study influences the sample size; a broad scope requires more subjects than does a study with a narrow scope.

_____ 3. Power analysis can be used to determine the sample size for the study.

_____ 4. The quality and the depth of information obtained from the study participants are used to determine the sample size.

_____ 5. As control in the study increases, the necessary sample size decreases.

_____ 6. The more sensitive the measurement methods used in a study, the fewer the subjects that are needed.

_____ 7. The more variables or concepts examined in a study, the larger the sample size that is needed.

_____ 8. The sample size needs to be large enough to prevent a Type II error.

_____ 9. Purposive sampling is a common method used to obtain an adequate sample size.

_____ 10. Simple random sampling is the strongest method of decreasing the potential for bias.

CROSSWORD PUZZLE

Directions: Complete the crossword puzzle below. Note that if the answer is more than one word, no blank spaces are left between the words.

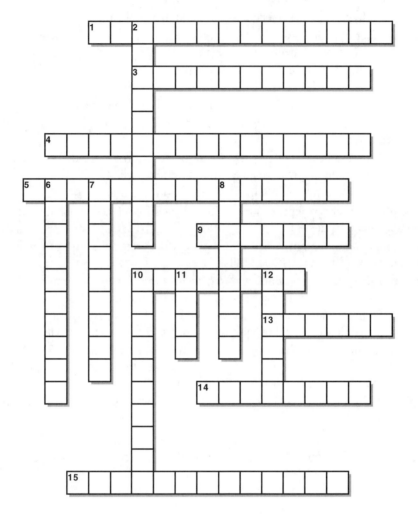

Across

1. Sample is _____ of the population
3. Random sampling
4. Group in a study
5. Used to select subjects
9. Possible sampling method used with studying subjects with HIV
10. People in a study
13. Equal opportunity to be a subject
14. Determines who is in a sample
15. Used to determine sample size

Down

2. Target _____
6. Population from which subjects are selected
7. Nonprobability sampling method
8. Make up the population
10. Number of subjects in a study
11. Slanted from truth
12. Population designated by sample criteria

EXERCISES IN CRITICAL APPRAISAL

Bindler, Massey, Shultz, Mills, and Short (2007) Study

Directions: Review the Bindler, Massey, Shultz, Mills, and Short (2007) study in Appendix B to answer the following questions.

1. Identify the study population. _____

2. List the sample criteria for this study. _____

   _____ .

   _____

   _____

   _____

   _____

3. Identify the sample characteristics for this study. _____

   _____

   _____

   _____

   _____

   _____

   _____

   _____

   _____

4. What is the sample size? _____

5. Was the sample size adequate? Provide a rationale. _____

   _____

   _____

   _____

   _____

   _____

6. What was the sample attrition for this study? Was this a study weakness? _____

_____

_____

_____

_____

_____

_____

_____

7. Was probability or nonprobability sampling used in this study? _____

8. What specific type of sampling method was used in this study? _____

9. Was the sample in this study representative of the target population studied? Provide a rationale.

_____

_____

_____

_____

_____

_____

_____

_____

10. Can the findings be generalized? Provide a rationale. _____

_____

_____

_____

_____

_____

_____

_____

_____

Padula, Yeaw, and Mistry (2009) Study

Directions: Review the Padula, Yeaw, and Mistry (2009) study in Appendix B to answer the following questions.

1. Identify the study populations. _____

2. List the sample criteria for this study. _____

    _____

    _____

    _____

    _____

    _____

    _____

3. Identify the sample characteristics for this study. _____

    _____

    _____

    _____

    _____

    _____

    _____

    _____

    _____

    _____

4. What number and percentage of the people screened did not meet the sample criteria? What number and percentage of the people screened met the sample criteria? What was the refusal rate?

    _____

    _____

    _____

    _____

    _____

    _____

5. What is the sample size? _____

6. Was the sample size adequate? Provide a rationale. _____

_____

_____

_____

_____

_____

7. What was the sample attrition for this study? _____

8. Was probability or nonprobability sampling used in this study? _____

9. What specific type of sampling method was used in this study? _____

10. Was the sample in this study representative of the target population studied? Provide a rationale.

_____

_____

_____

_____

_____

_____

11. Can the findings be generalized? Provide a rationale. _____

_____

_____

_____

_____

_____

_____

_____

Schachman (2010) Article

Directions: Review the Schachman (2010) article in Appendix B and answer the following questions.

1. Identify the study population. _____

2. List the sample criteria for this study. _____

_____

_____

_____

_____

_____

_____

_____

3. Identify the sample characteristics for this study. _____

_____

_____

_____

_____

_____

_____

_____

_____

_____

4. What is the sample size? _____ Was a power analysis done to determine sample size? Provide a rationale.

_____

_____

_____

5. Was the sample size adequate? Provide a rationale. _____

_____

_____

_____

_____

_____

6. What was the sample attrition for this study? _____

7. Was probability or nonprobability sampling used in this study? _____

8. What specific type of sampling method was used in this study? _____

9. Was the sample in this study representative of the population studied? Provide a rationale. _____

_____

_____

_____

_____

_____

_____

10. Can the findings be generalized? Provide a rationale. _____

_____

_____

_____

_____

_____

10 Clarifying Measurement and Data Collection in Quantitative Research

CHAPTER

INTRODUCTION

You need to read Chapter 10 and then complete the following exercises. These exercises will assist you in learning key terms and identifying and critically appraising measurement and data collection procedures in published studies. The answers for these exercises are in Appendix A under Chapter 10.

KEY TERMS

Measurement Concepts and Methods

Directions: Match each term below with its correct definition. Each term is used only once and all terms are defined.

a. Direct measurement
b. Indirect measurement
c. Interval-scale measurement
d. Interview
e. Likert scale
f. Measurement error
g. Nominal-scale measurement
h. Ordinal-scale measurement

i. Random measurement error
j. Ratio-scale measurement
k. Reliability
l. Structured observational measurement
m. Systematic measurement error
n. Validity
o. Visual analog scale

Definitions

_____ 1.   Lowest level of measurement when data can be organized into categories that are exclusive and exhaustive but the categories cannot be rank-ordered.

_____ 2.   Error that occurs consistently in one direction, such as a scale that weighs everyone 4 pounds less than their true weight, that can alter study results, and must be minimized.

_____ 3.   Error that is the difference between the measurement and true value of a variable that is without a pattern.

_____ 4.   A multiple-item scale used to measure perceptions of a phenomenon in a study, such as a 20-item scale used to measure perception of pain with ratings of 1—strongly disagree, 2—disagree, 3—agree, and 4—strongly agree.

_____ 5.   Consistency of the measurement technique.

_____ 6.   Level of measurement with categories that can be rank-ordered, such as levels of functional status—poor functional status, average functional status, and good functional status.

_____ 7.   A scale that uses a 100-mm line for a subject to mark that indicates the placement of his or her score.

_____ 8.   Measurement of a concrete variable (i.e., blood pressure) involves this type of measurement.

_____ 9.   Questions posed orally to a study participant as a way of collecting data.

____ 10. Level of measurement with equal intervals but without an absolute zero.

____ 11. Measurement of an abstract idea (i.e., anxiety) involves this type of measurement.

____ 12. How well the instrument measures what it is supposed to measure.

____ 13. Difference between the true measure and the actual measure.

____ 14. Level of measurement with equal intervals and an absolute zero point.

____ 15. Measurement method that requires observation of specific elements in a situation.

Data Collection

Directions: Match each term below with its correct definition. Each term is used only once and all terms are defined.

a. Computerized data collection   d. Data collection plan

b. Data collection   e. Data collection problems

c. Data collection form   f. Serendipity

Definitions

____ 1. Detailed plan of how the study will be implemented that is specific to the study being conducted and requires consideration of the commonplace elements of research.

____ 2. The actual process of selecting subjects and gathering data from these subjects by the researchers.

____ 3. Form that is developed or modified by the researcher, which is used for recording data.

____ 4. Concerns or issues that develop as data are collected and might include concerns with people, researchers, institutions, and events.

____ 5. The accidental discovery of something useful or valuable during the conduct of a study.

____ 6. Use of the microcomputer to collect large amounts of data with few errors that can be readily analyzed with a variety of statistical software packages.

KEY IDEAS

Directions: Fill in the blanks in this section with the appropriate word(s) or response(s).

1. A fasting blood sugar is an example of _____ measurement.

2. A reliability value of _____ is considered to be the lowest acceptable coefficient for a well-developed measurement tool.

3. In nominal measurement, the categories must be _____ and _____.

4. Ordinal data have _____ intervals, whereas interval data have _____ intervals.

5. A scale examining a participant's perception of anxiety with a 15-item scale with the possible responses to each item include "strongly disagree" through "strongly agree" would be a _____ scale.

6. If one IV bag has twice as much fluid as another, this would be measured using _____ level of measurement.

7. The coefficient for perfect reliability is _____.

8. A newly _____ tool can have a reliability of 0.70.

9. The common analysis conducted to determine homogeneity reliability of a scale that has measurement at least at the interval level is the _____.

10. If a study's measurement is not reliable **it is** or **it is not** valid? (Circle the correct response.)

11. When critically appraising the measurement section of a study, you need to check for information about the _____ and _____ of a scale.

12. A(n) _____ interview uses broad questions.

13. A(n) _____ interview is designed with specific questions to be asked by the researcher and is similar to a questionnaire.

14. Which has a higher response rate? (Circle one.) Mailed Questionnaire or Personal Interview

15. Questionnaires are used to make sure that there is _____ in data collection from subject to subject.

16. FACES scale used to measure perception of pain in children is a(n) _____ scale.

17. A scale 100 mm long used to measure anxiety is a(n) _____ scale.

18. Describe three situations that might result in error in the measurement of study variables.

    a. _____

    b. _____

    c. _____

19. List five tasks of the researcher during data collection.

    a. _____

    b. _____

    c. _____

    d. _____

    e. _____

20. _____ is the accidental discovery of useful information.

MAKING CONNECTIONS

Measurement Error

Directions: Match the type of measurement error likely to occur with the measurement method.

a. Random error
b. Systematic error

____ 1. Community income using a white, middle-class sample.
____ 2. Severity of cancer at diagnosis in a community, using patients in a county hospital.
____ 3. Average body weight measured at work at noon.
____ 4. Blood pressure taken with equipment that consistently measures the blood pressure low.
____ 5. Scores on drug calculation tests taken in the morning in a classroom.

Levels of Measurement

Directions: Match the level of measurement with the variables or measures listed below. You may use the categories more than once.

a. Nominal   c. Interval
b. Ordinal   d. Ratio

Variables

____ 1. Temperature
____ 2. Gender
____ 3. Educational level
____ 4. Final exam grade of 90%
____ 5. Type of cancer
____ 6. Severity of illness rank
____ 7. Score from visual analog scale
____ 8. Diagnosis of dyslipidemia
____ 9. Amount of stress measured with a Likert scale
____ 10. Height
____ 11. Percentage of weight gain
____ 12. Hemoglobin level
____ 13. Pain level ranking
____ 14. Apgar score
____ 15. Systolic and diastolic blood pressure
____ 16. Years of work experience
____ 17. Percentile score on an exam
____ 18. Hospital vs. hospice
____ 19. Salary ranges
____ 20. Marital status

Scales

Directions: Identify the type of scale being presented in the following examples.

a. Likert scale
b. Rating scale
c. Visual analog scale

____ 1.   I am satisfied with my nursing education: Agree   Neutral   Disagree
____ 2.   No Pain |_____| Most Severe Pain Possible
____ 3.   On a scale of 1 to 10, how much stress are you feeling?

Sensitivity and Specificity

Directions: Complete the other three cells in the table below.

1.

Diagnostic Test Results	Disease Present	Disease Not Present or Absent
Positive Test	*a* (true positive)	
Negative Test		

2. What is the formula for sensitivity? _____

3. What is the formula for specificity? _____

Sensitivity and Specificity of Colonoscopy Screening Tests

Diagnostic Test Results	Disease Present	Disease Not Present or Absent
Positive Test	90%	
Negative Test		85%

4. What is the percentage of false positive for the colonoscopy screening test using the data in the table above?

_____

5. What is the percentage of false negative for the colonoscopy screening test? _____

6. What is the sensitivity of the colonoscopy screening test? _____

7. What is the specificity of the colonoscopy screening test? _____

CROSSWORD PUZZLE

Directions: Complete the crossword puzzle below. Note: If the answer is more than one word, no blank spaces are left between the words.

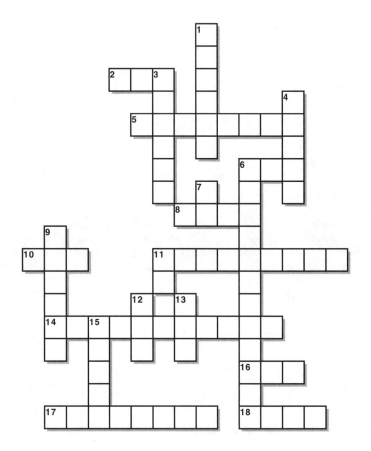

Across

2. Type of grain in cereal
5. _____ differential scale
6. Web address
8. Two felines
10. Opposite of "her"
11. Asking participant questions
14. Consistency of a measurement is called _____
16. Color of Santa's suit
17. Reflection of how well a measurement mirrors the concept of being measured
18. Proves ownership of a home

Down

1. _____ analog scale
3. Framework for a study
4. Numbered measurement tool
6. Broad interview question
7. Musical scale of Do, _____
9. 1-5 scale
11. Neither gender (slang)
12. Fifth month
13. Uncontrolled facial movement
15. Nominal _____ of measurement

EXERCISES IN CRITICAL APPRAISAL

Directions: Review the quantitative research articles in Appendix B and answer the following questions in the spaces provided.

Bindler, Massey, Shultz, Mills, and Short (2007) Study

Review the measurement section in Bindler, Massey, Shultz, Mills, and Short (2007) study and address the following critical appraisal questions.

1. Using the following table, identify the measurement method for selected variables in the Bindler et al. (2007) study. Also indicate whether the measurement method is a direct or indirect method of measuring the study variables.

Variable(s)	Measurement Method(s)	Direct or Indirect Measurement Method
Glucose		
TC, HDL-C, LDL-C		
Blood pressure		
Smoking history		
Body fat		
Diet		

2. Identify the precision and accuracy information for the following measurement methods.

Variable(s) and Measurement Methods	Precision and Accuracy Information from Study
Glucose: Blood draw	
Blood pressure: Cuff, stethoscope, and sphygmomanometer	

3. Critically appraise the quality of the measurement of glucose and blood pressure._____

_____

_____

_____

_____

_____

_____

_____

_____

_____

4. Identify the validity and reliability of the YAQ used to measure diet and the questionnaire used to measure smoking history in the table below.

Diet: YAQ Questionnaire	
Smoking History Questionnaire	

5. Critically appraise the reliability and the validity of the YAQ and smoking history questionnaires.

_____

_____

_____

_____

_____

_____

_____

_____

6. Describe the data collection process for the Bindler et al. (2007) study._____

_____

_____

_____

_____

_____

_____

_____

_____

_____

_____

7. Critically appraise the quality of the data collection process in the Bindler et al. study._____

_____

_____

_____

_____

_____

_____

_____

_____

_____

_____

Padula, Yeaw, and Mistry (2009) Study

Directions: Review the measurement section in Padula, Yeaw, and Mistry (2009) study and address the following critical appraisal questions.

1. Using the following table, identify the measurement method for selected variables in the Padula et al. (2009) study. Also indicate whether the measurement method is a direct or indirect method of measuring the study variables.

Variable(s)	Measurement Method(s)	Direct or Indirect Measurement Method
Inspiratory muscle strength (IMS)		
Self-efficacy		

2. Identify the precision and accuracy information for the following measurement method.

Variable(s) and Measurement Methods	Precision and Accuracy Information from Study
Inspiratory muscle strength (IMS): measured by PI_{max}	

3. Critically appraise the quality of the measurement of IMS._____

_____

_____

_____

_____

_____

_____

4. Identify the validity and reliability of the chronic obstructive pulmonary disease (COPD) self-efficacy scale (CSES) used to measure self-efficacy in HF patients in the table below.

Scale	Reliability and Validity Information from the Study
CSES	

5. Critically appraise the reliability and the validity of the CSES. _____

_____

_____

_____

_____

_____

_____

_____

_____

6. Describe the data collection process for the Padula et al. (2009) study. _____

_____

_____

_____

_____

_____

_____

_____

7. Critically appraise the quality of the data collection process in the Padula et al. study. _____

_____

_____

_____

_____

_____

_____

11 Understanding Statistics in Research

INTRODUCTION

You need to read Chapter 11 and then complete the following exercises. These exercises will assist you in learning key terms and identifying and critically appraising statistical techniques, results, and discussion sections in published studies. The answers to these exercises are in Appendix A under Chapter 11.

KEY TERMS

Directions: Match each term below with its correct definition. Each term is used only once and all terms are defined.

a. Alpha
b. Confirmatory analysis
c. Decision theory
d. Dependent groups
e. Effect size
f. Findings
g. Generalization
h. Implications for nursing
i. Independent groups
j. Outliers
k. Post hoc analysis
l. Power
m. Probability theory
n. Type I error
o. Type II error

Definitions

_____ 1.   Acceptance of the null hypothesis when it is false.
_____ 2.   The probability that a statistical test will detect a significant difference or relationship that exists.
_____ 3.   Findings acquired from a specific study are applied to a target population.
_____ 4.   Rejection of the null hypothesis when it is true.
_____ 5.   Indicates the strength of a relationship between two variables.
_____ 6.   The likelihood of an event occurring in a given situation.
_____ 7.   Theory applied when testing for differences between groups with the assumption that the groups are from the same population, so they are not different.
_____ 8.   Subjects with extreme values.
_____ 9.   Level of significance that is set at the start of a study.
_____ 10. Changes that should be made in practice, based on the findings.
_____ 11. Results from data analysis are translated into _____.
_____ 12. Persons in control groups matched to the experimental groups.
_____ 13. Groups selected so the participants are unrelated to the selection of other subjects.
_____ 14. Data analysis guided by study objectives, questions, or hypotheses.
_____ 15. Data analysis after an analysis of variance (ANOVA) to determine differences among three groups.

KEY IDEAS

Directions: Fill in the blanks in this section with the appropriate word(s) or response(s).

1. List five types of results from quasi-experimental and experimental study results.

    a. _____

    b. _____

    c. _____

    d. _____

    e. _____

2. Identify the six areas included in the discussion section of a research report.

    a. _____

    b. _____

    c. _____

    d. _____

    e. _____

    f. _____

3. List four parts of the data analysis process:

    a. _____

    b. _____

    c. _____

    d. _____

4. The purpose of statistical analysis is to _____.

5. List three statistical analysis techniques used to describe the sample.

    a. _____

    b. _____

    c. _____

6. Draw and label a normal curve with a mean of 0 and a standard deviation of 1.

7. In a normal distribution of scores, what percent of the scores fall between –1.96 and +1.96 standard deviations of the mean? _____

8. The most precise level of statistical significance is achieved by conducting a **one-** or **two-tailed** level of significance? (Circle correct answer.)

9. A Type _____ error occurs if you say that a therapeutic touch intervention works to relieve acute pain when it does not.

10. The abbreviation for analysis of variance is _____.

11. The measure of central tendency calculated for nominal level data is _____.

12. What does "*n*" represent in a statistical table? _____.

13. A distribution of data that is asymmetrical because of outliers is called _____.

14. A diagram of points placed at their relative scores along a best fit line is called a(n) _____ _____.

15. Data analysis that is conducted on two variables is called _____.

MAKING CONNECTIONS

Linking Statistics with Analysis Techniques

Directions: Match each statistic with its appropriate analysis technique. Each statistic is used only once and all analysis techniques have a statistic included.

Statistics

a. *df*

b. *SD*

c. *r*

d. *ES*

e. *R10*

f. *F*

g. χ^2

h. %

i. *t*

j. α

Analysis Techniques

____ 1. Standard deviation

____ 2. Regression analysis

_____ 3.   Alpha

_____ 4.   Pearson product moment correlation

_____ 5.   Analysis of variance

_____ 6.   Degrees of freedom

_____ 7.   Effect size

_____ 8.   Chi-square

_____ 9.   Percentage

_____ 10.   *t*-test

Linking Level of Measurement with Analysis Techniques

Directions: Link the appropriate level of measurement for data to be analyzed by the following analysis techniques. The levels of measurement can be used more than once. Some of the statistical analyses can be used for two different levels of measurement.

Level of Measurement for Data

a.   Nominal level

b.   Ordinal level

c.   Interval/ratio level

Statistical Analysis Techniques

_____ 1.   *t*-test for independent groups

_____ 2.   Chi-square

_____ 3.   Mean

_____ 4.   Pearson product moment correlation

_____ 5.   Percentages

_____ 6.   Median

_____ 7.   Regression analysis

_____ 8.   Effect size

_____ 9.   Standard deviation

_____ 10.   Range

_____ 11.   Mode

_____ 12.   Ungrouped frequencies

_____ 13.   Analysis of variance

_____ 14.   *t*-test for dependent groups

_____ 15.   Grouped frequencies

Statements, Inferences, and Generalizations

Directions: Match the statement categories with its sample study. You may use the categories more than once.

Statement Categories

a. Decision theory statement
b. Probability theory statement

c. Inference
d. Generalization

Example Studies

_____ 1. The experimental pain assessment tool can be used to successfully assess pain levels in hospitalized patients after many different types of surgery.

_____ 2. This suggests that when stress occurs, probably disruption in social activity is likely to occur.

_____ 3. No significant differences were found in functional outcomes between the two groups of patients treated with sterile petroleum gauze or sterile nonmedicated gauze.

_____ 4. Because most major risk factors thought to affect mental health did not change, and no adverse changes in sleepiness were observed during the intervention period, it is plausible to argue that the group discussion would not have reduced insomnia reports over longer time periods.

_____ 5. The results of this study indicated that community instruction regarding choking can aid in decreasing admissions to the hospital for choking. Written instructions with pictures, understandable on an elementary-grade reading level, appear to be successful in the teaching and learning of measures to alleviate choking episodes in the home and community.

_____ 6. Automatic defibrillators can be used safely for cases of cardiac arrest in the community.

Describing the Sample

Directions: Referring to the table below, answer the following questions in the spaces provided.

Nurses (N = 100)	Frequency (f)	Percentage (%)
Age in Years		
18-29	10	10%
30-39	20	20%
40-49	35	35%
50-59	30	30%
60 and greater	5	5%
Nursing Education		
Associate Degree in Nursing (ADN)	50	50%
Diploma	20	20%
Bachelors' of Science in Nursing (BSN)	30	30%

1. Which variable contains grouped data? _____

2. What is the mode of "Nursing Education?" _____

3. What is the median "Age Group?" _____

Measures of Central Tendency

Directions: Referring to the results of a 10-item Likert scale with response options of 1-5, printed below, answer the following questions in the spaces provided.

mean = 3.42 $SD = 0.76$

median = 3.10   mode = 3.00

1.   Which value is the average? _____
2.   Which value is the 50th percentile? _____
3.   What does the mode represent? _____
4.   Using the *SD* value, what is the range of values ± 1 *SD* from the mean? _____

Name That Statistical Test!

Directions: Match the following statistical test findings with their test names. Then give the definition of each of the tests and the level of data (i.e., nominal, ordinal, interval, ratio) appropriately used for each.

Statistical Test Findings

a. $\chi^2 = 4.61$ $df = 2$ $p = 0.10$
b. $t = 15.631$ $df = 180$ $p = 0.001$
c. $r = -0.315$ $df = 76$ $p < 0.05$
d. $F = 56.71$ $df = 8120$ $p < 0.001$

Test Names   **Purpose**   **Level of Data**

____ 1. ANOVA _____

_____

____ 2. Chi-square _____

_____

____ 3. Pearson product moment correlation _____

_____

____ 4. *t*-test _____

_____

Significance of Results

Directions: In the following statistical findings, indicate whether the results were statistically significant (*) or not statistically significant (NS), assuming a level of significance set at alpha = 0.05. You may use each category more than once.

* = Statistically Significant   **NS = Not Statistically Significant**

____ 1. $\chi^2 = 1.61$ $df = 2$ $p = 0.10$
____ 2. $t = 15.631$ $df = 180$ $p = 0.001$
____ 3. $r = -0.315$ $df = 76$ $p < 0.05$
____ 4. $F = 1.37$ $df = 25$ $p = 0.23$

CROSSWORD PUZZLE

Directions: Complete the crossword puzzle below. Note: If the answer is more than one word, no blank spaces are left between the words.

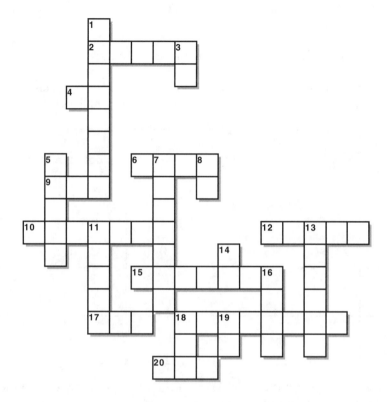

Across

2. Short for analysis of variance
4. Roman numeral for 11
6. Choose government leader by _____
9. _____, two, three
10. Measure of _____ tendency
12. 18 – 25
15. Word for "%"
17. Opposite of "bottom"
18. Practical significance
20. Four, five, _____, seven

Down

1. Analysis of _____
3. Article used for noun starting with vowel
5. The strength of a statistical test to detect differences
7. Extreme score
8. Abbreviation for "emergency room"
11. $t = 3.48$ $df = 20$ $p = 0.001$
13. _____ distribution
14. Us
16. Two _____ed test
18. _____-square
19. _____, ego, superego

EXERCISES IN CRITICAL APPRAISAL

Bindler, Massey, Shultz, Mills, and Short (2007) Study

Directions: Read the Bindler, Massey, Schultz, Mills, and Short (2007) study found in Appendix B and then answer the following questions in the spaces provided.

1. How many groups did this study have and what were the names of the groups?_____

2. For each variable in the table, indicate the level of measurement (i.e., nominal, ordinal, interval, or ratio) and the descriptive analysis technique(s) that were conducted in the Bindler et al. (2007) study.

Demographic and Study Variables	Level of Measurement	Descriptive Analysis Techniques
Gender		
Age in years		
Family history of overweight		
Systolic blood pressure		

3. What was the mean insulin value in the study? Were the insulin values significantly different for the ethnic groups? Which ethnic group had the highest mean insulin value?

_____

_____

_____

_____

_____

_____

_____

_____

_____

4. What were the results for Research Question 4: "Which data predict insulin levels in this multiethnic sample of children?" What analysis technique was used to obtain these results?

_____

_____

_____

_____

_____

_____

_____

_____

_____

5. What were the limitations of the Bindler et al. (2007) study? Should the study findings be generalized based on these limitations?

_____

_____

_____

_____

_____

_____

_____

_____

_____

_____

_____

Padula, Yeaw, and Mistry (2009) Study

Directions: Read the Padula, Yeaw, and Mistry (2009) study found in Appendix B and then answer the following questions in the spaces provided.

1. For each variable in the table, indicate the level of measurement (i.e., nominal, ordinal, interval, or ratio) and the descriptive analysis technique(s) that were conducted in the Padula et al. (2009) study.

Demographic Variables	Level of Measurement	Descriptive Analysis Techniques
Marital status		
New York Heart Association Classification		
Age in years		
Mean heart rate		

2. Was the maximal inspiratory pressure (PI_{max}) significantly different for the treatment group versus the control group? What was the result, and what analysis technique was used to obtain this result?

_____

_____

_____

_____

_____

_____

_____

_____

3. Was there a significant difference between the treatment and control groups on physical/functional and psychosocial health related quality of life (HRQOL) and self-efficacy? Provide a rationale for these results.

_____

_____

_____

_____

_____

_____

_____

_____

_____

4. What are the clinical implications discussed in this study? _____

_____

_____

_____

_____

_____

_____

_____

_____

_____

_____

_____

5. What are some of the recommendations for future research? _____

_____

_____

_____

_____

_____

_____

_____

_____

_____

CHAPTER 12

Critical Appraisal of Quantitative and Qualitative Research for Nursing Practice

INTRODUCTION

You need to read Chapter 12 and then complete the following exercises. These exercises will assist you in understanding the quantitative and qualitative research critical appraisal processes. The answers to these exercises are in Appendix A under Chapter 12.

KEY TERMS

Directions: Match each term with its correct definition. Each term is used only once and all terms are defined.

a. Analysis phase of critical appraisal
b. Comparison phase of critical appraisal
c. Comprehension phase of critical appraisal
d. Critical appraisal of qualitative research
e. Evaluation step of critical appraisal
f. Intellectual critical appraisal of a study

Definitions

____ 1. Careful, complete examination of a study to judge the strengths and weaknesses of the study, credibility of the study findings, and the usefulness of the findings for practice.

____ 2. Critical appraisal step in which the ideal for each step of the quantitative research process is compared with the real steps in a published study.

____ 3. Critical appraisal step for quantitative research that involves determining the strengths and limitations of the logical links connecting one study element with another.

____ 4. Critical appraisal step during which the reader gains understanding of the terms in the research report; identifies the study elements; and grasps the nature, significance, and meaning of these elements.

____ 5. Critical appraisal of a quantitative study in which the reader examines the meaning and significance of a study according to set criteria and compares it with previous studies conducted in the area and determines the significance of the findings for nursing practice.

____ 6. Rigorous and comprehensive review of the quality and credibility of a qualitative study.

KEY IDEAS

Directions: Fill in the blanks with the appropriate word(s).

1. An intellectual research critical appraisal involves careful examination of all aspects of a study to judge the
   _____, _____, _____
   _____, and _____ of the study.

2. Identify three important questions that are part of an intellectual research critical appraisal.

   a. _____

   b. _____

   c. _____

3. Describe your role in conducting research critical appraisals. _____

   _____

   _____

   _____

   _____

   _____

   _____

4. List the four steps of the quantitative research critical appraisal process.

   a. _____

   b. _____

   c. _____

   d. _____

5. Adherence to ethical standards in qualitative research involves protecting participants'
   _____ and obtaining _____ from the partici-
   pants.

6. Qualitative research is based on a philosophical perspective that is called the _____
   _____.

7. In qualitative research, the use of focus groups, interviews, and observation is part of _____
   _____.

8. In general, qualitative studies are founded in an interpretive paradigm and methods of naturalistic inquiry
   that is referred to as the _____.

MAKING CONNECTIONS

Directions: Match the steps of the quantitative research critical appraisal process with the examples provided.

a. Analysis
b. Comparison
c. Comprehension
d. Evaluation

_____ 1. Identify the study framework.

_____ 2. Is the study feasible to conduct in terms of the money commitment; researchers' expertise; availability of subjects, facility, and equipment; and ethical considerations?

_____ 3. Identify the methods of measurement used in the study.

_____ 4. Do the findings add to the current body of knowledge?

_____ 5. Is the design linked to the sampling method, study instruments, and statistical analyses?

_____ 6. Do the data analyses address the study purpose and the research objectives, questions, or hypotheses?

_____ 7. Is the treatment clearly described and consistently implemented?

_____ 8. To what populations can the findings be generalized?

_____ 9. Are the physiological measures used in a study accurate, precise, selective, and sensitive?

_____ 10. Was the purpose identified in the study?

EXERCISES IN CRITICAL APPRAISAL

Directions: Read the research articles in Appendix B. Conduct the steps of the quantitative research critical appraisal process (comprehension, comparison, analysis, and evaluation) on two of the studies. Conduct the qualitative research critical appraisal process on one of the studies. Use the quantitative and qualitative critical appraisal guidelines provided in Chapter 12, Critical Appraisal of Quantitative and Qualitative Research for Nursing Practice, in your textbook.

1. Conduct a critical appraisal of the Bindler, Massey, Shultz, Mills, and Short (2007) article using the guidelines outlined in your text. Many parts of this study were critically appraised in Chapters 1 through 11 of this study guide.
   a. Conduct the comprehension step of the critical appraisal process. Questions are outlined in your text to direct your critical appraisal.
   b. Do a critical appraisal that includes the comparison, analysis, and evaluation steps of the quantitative research critical appraisal process.

2. Conduct a critical appraisal of the Padula, Yeaw, and Mistry (2009) article using the guidelines outlined in your text. Many parts of this study were critically appraised in Chapters 1 though 11 of this study guide.
   a. Conduct the comprehension step of the critical appraisal process. Questions are outlined in your text to direct this process.
   b. Do a critical appraisal that includes the comparison, analysis, and evaluation steps of the quantitative research critical appraisal process.

3. Conduct a critical appraisal of the Schachman (2010) article using the qualitative critical appraisal guidelines outlined in Chapter 12 of your text.

13 Building an Evidence-Based Nursing Practice

INTRODUCTION

You need to read Chapter 13 and then complete the following exercises. These exercises will assist you in understanding the process of developing an evidence-based practice in nursing. The answers to these exercises are in Appendix A under Chapter 13.

KEY TERMS

Directions: Match each term with its definition or description. Each term is used only once and all terms are defined.

Terms

a. Algorithms
b. Best research evidence
c. Evidence-based practice
d. Evidence-based practice centers
e. Evidence-based guidelines
f. Grove Model for Implementing Evidence-Based Guidelines in Practice
g. Integrative review of research
h. Iowa Model of Evidence-Based Practice
i. Meta-analysis
j. PICO format
k. Qualitative research synthesis
l. Stetler Model of Research Utilization to Facilitate Evidence-Based Practice
m. Systematic review
n. Translation research

Definitions

_____ 1. A structured, comprehensive synthesis of quantitative studies in a particular health care area to determine the best research evidence available for expert clinicians to use to promote evidence-based practice.

_____ 2. Review initiated by a clinical question that includes the following elements: population of interest, intervention needed for practice, comparison of interventions to determine best practice, and outcomes needed for practice.

_____ 3. A process of statistically pooling the results from previous studies into a single quantitative analysis that provides a high level of evidence for an intervention's efficacy.

_____ 4. Highest quality research knowledge produced by the conduct and synthesis of numerous high-quality studies in a health-related area.

_____ 5. Patient care guidelines that are based on synthesized research findings from systematic reviews, meta-analyses, integrative reviews of research, and extensive clinical trials; supported by consensus from recognized national experts; and affirmed by outcomes obtained by clinicians.

_____ 6. A process that includes the identification, analysis, and synthesis of research findings from independent quantitative and sometimes qualitative studies to determine the current knowledge (what is known and not known) in a particular area.

____ 7.   This is a comprehensive framework to enhance the use of research findings by nurses that includes the phases of preparation, validation, comparative evaluation/decision making, translation/application, and evaluation.

____ 8.   Model developed by one of the textbook authors to promote the use of evidence-based guidelines in practice.

____ 9.   Centers designated by the Agency for Healthcare Research and Quality for the development of research in designated areas and the translation of the evidence-based research findings into clinical practice.

____ 10.   A process and product of systematically reviewing and formally integrating the findings from qualitative studies.

____ 11.   A model developed by Titler and colleagues in 1994 and revised in 2001 that provides direction for the development of evidence-based practice in a clinical agency.

____ 12.   A practice that involves the conscientious integration of best research evidence with clinical expertise and patient values and needs in the delivery of quality, cost-effective health care.

____ 13.   Clinical decision-making trees or figures nurses use when implementing research evidence in practice.

____ 14.   New and evolving type of research that is defined by the National Institutes of Health (NIH) as the translation of basic scientific discoveries into practical applications.

KEY IDEAS

Directions: Fill in the blanks or provide the appropriate responses.

1.   List three reasons nursing needs to develop an evidence-based practice.

   a.   _____

   b.   _____

   c.   _____

2.   Identify three sources you might access to keep current with the research literature.

   a.   _____

   b.   _____

   c.   _____

3.   Identify two barriers or criticisms of evidence-based practice in nursing.

   a.   _____

   b.   _____

4.   Identify two reasons why nursing lacks the research evidence needed for implementing an evidence-based practice.

   a.   _____

   b.   _____

5. Identify and describe three ways that research findings might be implemented in nursing practice that were discussed in Stetler's Model of Research Utilization to Facilitate Evidence-Based Practice.

a. _____

Description: _____

_____

b. _____

Description: _____

_____

c. _____

Description: _____

_____

6. Identify two sources of summaries of nursing research knowledge.

a. _____

b. _____

7. Identify the five phases of the Stetler Model of Research Utilization to Facilitate Evidence-Based Practice.

a. _____

b. _____

c. _____

d. _____

e. _____

8. The comparative evaluation phase of Stetler's Model includes four parts: substantiating evidence, fit of the setting, _____, and _____.

9. Identify the three options of the decision-making phase of the Stetler's Model.

a. _____

b. _____

c. _____

10. The _____ Model was developed in 1994 and revised in 2001 to promote evidence-based practice in nursing.

11. The Joint National Committee on Prevention, Detection, Evaluation, and Treatment of High Blood Pressure (JNC VII) guideline that was published in 2003 is an example of _____.

12. The National Clearinghouse Guidelines (NCG) website was developed by the Agency for _____ _____and_____.

13. The NCG is maintained by a partnership with two organizations:

    a. _____

    b. _____

14. In 1997, the Agency for Healthcare Research and Quality established 12 _____ _____ Centers of excellence to promote the conduct of research and the development of evidence-based guidelines for practice.

15. The goal of the Grove Model for Implementing Evidence-Based Guidelines in Practice is _____.

16. NIH is developing funding awards for translational research to improve the _____ _____.

MAKING CONNECTIONS

Application of the Phases of Stetler's Model

Directions: Match the phase in Stetler's Model with the appropriate description and/or example.

Phase

a. Comparative evaluation/decision making
b. Evaluation
c. Preparation
d. Translation/application
e. Validation

Descriptions

_____ 1.   The phase in which nurses evaluate the feasibility of using the Braden scale to prevent pressure ulcers in their clinical agency.

_____ 2.   The phase in which nurses develop a formal protocol for treatment of stage IV pressure ulcers in older adults.

_____ 3.   The first awareness of the existence of an exercise program for severely disabled children obtained from attending a research conference and reading the study and similar studies in research journals.

_____ 4.   Research knowledge about prevention of hospitalized infections is synthesized and evaluated using specific criteria.

_____ 5.   The incidence of hospital-acquired infections is examined following the implementation of a new protocol to prevent infections.

Agency's Readiness for Evidence-Based Practice

Think about the clinical agency in which you are currently doing your clinical hours.

1. Are the agency's policies and nursing protocols based on research? Provide a rationale for your answer.

    _____

    _____

    _____

    _____

    _____

    _____

    _____

2. If you answered "no" to the previous question, what is the basis of the policies and protocols of your agency?

    _____

    _____

    _____

    _____

    _____

    _____

    _____

3. Who are the change agents or innovators in this agency? (Record only the persons' positions.)_____

    _____

    _____

4. Does the agency provide research publications for nurses? If so, provide some examples of these publications.

    _____

    _____

    _____

    _____

5. Does the agency have the goal of evidence-based practice? _____

_____

_____

_____

_____

_____

_____

_____

6. Is the agency seeking magnet status? What is the link of evidence-based practice to magnet status?

_____

_____

_____

_____

_____

_____

_____

_____

EXERCISES IN CRITICAL APPRAISAL

Read and critically appraise the systematic review of childhood obesity prevention developed by Wofford (2008) that is posted online in the 'Research Articles' section of the Evolve resources for Understanding Nursing Research *at http://evolve. elsevier.com/burns/understanding. The reference citation is:*

Wofford, L. G. (2008). Systematic review of childhood obesity prevention. *Journal of Pediatric Nursing, 23*(1), 5-19.

Use the following guidelines to conduct your critical appraisal.

Guidelines for Critically Appraising Systematic Reviews

1. Was the purpose (or objectives) of the review clearly stated? Provide a rationale. _____

_____

_____

_____

_____

_____

_____

2. Did the reviewers report a systematic and comprehensive search strategy to identify relevant studies?

_____

_____

_____

_____

_____

3. Were inclusion and exclusion criteria for studies reported and were they appropriate (i.e., was selection bias avoided)?

_____

_____

_____

_____

_____

_____

_____

_____

_____

4. Was the quality of included studies assessed appropriately?_____

_____

_____

_____

_____

_____

_____

_____

_____

5. Were the results of the included studies combined systematically and appropriately? _____

_____

_____

_____

_____

_____

_____

_____

_____

6. Were the conclusions supported by the data? (Craig & Smyth, 2007, p. 194). _____

_____

_____

_____

_____

_____

_____

Provide a summary of your critical appraisal of this systematic review. _____

_____

_____

_____

_____

_____

_____

_____

_____

_____

GOING BEYOND

1. Conduct a project to promote evidence-based practice in a selected area of your practice. Use the following steps as a guide.
    a. Identify a clinical problem that might be improved by using research knowledge.
    b. Locate and review the studies in this problem area.
    c. Summarize what is known and not known regarding this problem.
    d. Select a model or theory to direct your use of research evidence in practice, such as the Stetler's Model of Research Utilization to Facilitate Evidence-Based Practice or the Iowa Model of Evidence-Based Practice.
    e. Assess your agency's readiness to make the change.
    f. Communicate the evidence-based change proposed to the nursing personnel, other health professionals, and administration.
    g. Support those persons involved in making the evidence-based change in practice.
    h. Implement the evidence-based change by developing a protocol, algorithm, or policy to be used in practice.
    i. Develop evaluation strategies to determine the effect or outcomes of the evidence-based change on patient, provider, and agency.
    j. Evaluate over time to determine whether the evidence-based change should be continued. You might also extend the change to additional units or clinical agencies.

2. Use the Grove Model for Implementing Evidence-Based Guidelines to implement an evidence-based guideline from the Agency for Healthcare Research and Quality website in your practice.

CHAPTER 14

Introduction to Outcomes Research

INTRODUCTION

You need to read Chapter 14 and then complete the following exercises. These exercises will assist you in learning key terms and in reading and comprehending published outcomes studies. The answers for these exercises are in Appendix A under Chapter 14.

KEY TERMS

Directions: Match each term below with its correct definition. Each term is used only once and all terms are defined.

Terms

a. Clinical decision analysis
b. Consensus knowledge building
c. Cost-benefit analysis
d. Efficiency
e. Health (as defined by Donabedian)
f. Interdisciplinary team
g. Opportunity costs

h. Outcomes research
i. Out-of-pocket costs
j. Population-based study
k. Prospective cohort study
l. Research tradition
m. Standard of care

Definitions

_____ 1. Time and salary lost when families care for ill members.

_____ 2. Norm by which quality of care is judged. Clinical guidelines, critical paths, and care maps define these.

_____ 3. Type of research that focuses on the end results of patient care.

_____ 4. Members of health care team that includes nurses, physicians, therapists, social workers, respiratory therapists, pharmacists, and physical therapists.

_____ 5. The least costly method.

_____ 6. Defines an acceptable research methodology and is still emerging for outcomes research.

_____ 7. Conditions are studied in the context of the community rather than the medical system.

_____ 8. Multidisciplinary groups' agreement on the outcome.

_____ 9. Concept that has many aspects, such as physical-physiological function, psychological function, and social function that are examined in outcomes research.

_____ 10. Costs and benefits of alternatives, assessed in monetary terms.

_____ 11. Costs paid by the patient and/or family members that are not reimbursable by the insurance company.

_____ 12.   Systematic method of describing clinical problems, identifying possible diagnostic and management courses of action, assessing the probability and value of various outcomes, and then calculating the optimal course of action.

_____ 13.   Epidemiological study following people into the future who are identified as at risk for experiencing a particular event.

KEY IDEAS

Directions: Fill in the blanks in this section with the appropriate word(s) or response(s).

1.   Outcomes research focuses on _____.

2.   The meeting of which two National Institutes of Health (NIH) study sections ultimately led to the development of the Agency for Health Services Research (AHSR)?

   a.   _____

   b.   _____

3.   What was the first large-scale study to examine factors influencing patient outcomes? _____

   _____

4.   The Medical Outcomes Study (MOS) was flawed because it failed to control for the following three elements:

   a.   _____

   b.   _____

   c.   _____

5.   The following three components, commonly performed by nurses, were considered by MOS to be components of medical practice:

   a.   _____

   b.   _____

   c.   _____

6.   Clinical guideline panels were developed to: _____

   _____

   _____

7.   Examining the impact of nursing on overall hospital outcomes requires _____

   _____

8.   To evaluate an outcome, the outcomes must be clearly linked to the process that caused the

   _____.

9. List three examples of standards of care:

    a. _____

    b. _____

    c. _____

10. _____ samples are preferred in outcome studies.

11. To allow evaluation or monitoring of individual patient care, the following information must be available in large databases:

    a. _____

    b. _____

    c. _____

    d. _____

12. From an outcomes research perspective, identify three questions that might be asked about interventions:

    a. _____

    b. _____

    c. _____

13. Treatment matching is used when the following conditions are met:

    a. _____

    b. _____

    c. _____

14. Outcomes selected for nursing studies should be those that are _____
    _____.

15. Instruments for outcomes studies should be selected for their sensitivity to _____
    _____.

16. The Nursing's Safety and Quality Initiative was developed by _____.

17. In analyzing improvement of patients' treatment with a particular intervention, the following parameters should be reported:

    a. _____

    b. _____

    c. _____

    d. _____

    e. _____

18. List two nursing classification schemes:

a. _____

b. _____

19. In analysis of improvement, the _____ of persons who improved must be calculated.

20. Providing results of outcomes studies to others is called _____.

MAKING CONNECTIONS

Research Strategies for Outcomes Studies

Directions: Match the outcomes research design with its example study.

Research Designs

a. Consensus knowledge building

b. Prospective cohort studies

c. Retrospective cohort studies

d. Population-based studies

e. Clinical decision analysis

f. Study of effectiveness of interdisciplinary teams

g. Economic studies

Example Studies

____ 1. Studying how antihypertensive drugs are prescribed for older women.

____ 2. Gathering data on the exposure to benzene in people living near a toxic waste dump.

____ 3. Costs of drugs and prescribing habits of primary care providers.

____ 4. Communication patterns between nurses and physical therapists.

____ 5. Multidisciplinary groups present outcomes findings on nutrition at a conference.

____ 6. Monitoring the development of asthma in children whose school is next to a truck stop.

____ 7. Following women at risk for developing skin cancer over 20 years.

Major Contributors to Outcomes Research

Directions: Match the acronyms with their full names, and then describe in the spaces provided each of their contributions to outcomes research.

Acronyms

a. AHRQ

b. ANA

c. NDNQI

d. NINR

e. NIC

Contributors and Descriptions

1. National Institute for Nursing Research:_____

2. National Database of Nursing Quality Indicators: _____

3. American Nurses Association:_____

4. Agency for Healthcare Research and Quality:_____

5. Nursing Interventions Classification:_____

EXERCISES IN CRITICAL APPRAISAL

Directions: Read the Kanak, Titler, Shever, Fei, Dochterman, and Picone (2008) article found in the 'Research Articles' section of the Evolve resources for Understanding Nursing Research *at http://evolve.elsevier.com/burns/understanding. The citation for this article is:*

Kanak, M. F., Titler, M., Shever, L., Fei, Q., Dochterman, J., & Picone, D. M. (2008). The effects of hospitalization on multiple units. *Applied Nursing Research*, *21*(1), 15-22.

Answer the following questions related to this study.

1. What type of study is the Kanak et al. (2008) study? Give a rationale for your answer. _____

_____

_____

_____

_____

_____

2. What outcomes were being considered in this study? _____

_____

_____

_____

_____

_____

_____

_____

_____

_____

_____

_____

_____

3. What was the design for this study? _____

_____

_____

_____

_____

_____

4. What were the key findings from this study? _____

_____

_____

_____

_____

_____

_____

_____

_____

_____

_____

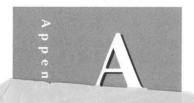

Answers to Study Guide Exercises

CHAPTER 1—INTRODUCTION TO NURSING RESEARCH AND EVIDENCE-BASED PRACTICE

Key Terms

Acquiring Knowledge and Research Methods

1.	g	9.	l
2.	h	10.	d
3.	e	11.	i
4.	j	12.	k
5.	m	13.	a
6.	b	14.	o
7.	c	15.	n
8.	f		

Evidence-Based Practice Terms

1. e
2. b
3. a
4. d
5. c

Processes Used to Synthesize Research Evidence

1. e
2. c
3. a
4. d
5. b

Key Ideas

How Research Influences Practice

1. Description involves identifying the nature and attributes of nursing phenomena. Descriptive knowledge generated through research can be used to identify what exists in nursing practice, to discover new information, and to classify information of use in the discipline. For example, describing those who are at risk for HIV, identifying the signs and symptoms for making a nursing diagnosis, and describing the spread of the H1N1 flu.
2. Explanation focuses on clarifying relationships among variables or identifying the reasons certain events occur. For example, risk for developing pressure ulcers is related to level of mobility and age; as mobility decreases and age increases, pressure ulcer risk increases.
3. Prediction involves estimating the probability of a specific outcome in a given situation. With predictive knowledge, nurses can anticipate the effects nursing interventions would have on patients and families; for

example, predicting the effects of a long-term exercise program on women with breast cancer. Predictive knowledge also could predict the effect of nutrition and exercise on obesity in children and adults.

4. Control is the ability to manipulate a situation to produce the desired outcome. Thus nurses could prescribe certain interventions to help patients and families achieve quality outcomes. For example, you would prescribe the use of warm, not cold, applications for the resolution of normal saline IV infiltrations. Back massage might be prescribed as a treatment for high blood pressure.

Historical Events Influencing Nursing Research

1. Nightingale
2. 1952
3. Sigma Theta Tau
4. You might list any three of the following journals:
    Research in Nursing & Health
    Western Journal of Nursing Research
    Scholarly Inquiry for Nursing Practice
    Applied Nursing Research
    Nursing Science Quarterly
5. integrative reviews of research or summaries of current research knowledge in the areas of nursing practice, nursing care delivery, nursing education, and the nursing profession
6. 1985
7. National Institute for Nursing Research (NINR)
8. conduct, support, and dissemination of information
9. "The mission for NINR for the 21st century is to promote and improve the health of individuals, families, communities, and populations. NINR supports and conducts clinical and basic research and research training on health and illness across the lifespan. The research focus encompasses health promotion and disease prevention, quality of life, health disparities, and end-of-life. NINR seeks to extend nursing science by integrating the biological and behavioral sciences, employing new technologies to research questions, improving research methods, and developing the scientists of the future" (NINR website: http://www.ninr.nih.gov/AboutNINR/NINRMissionandStrategicPlan/, 2010).
10. clinical
11. Agency for Health Care Policy and Research (AHCPR)
12. Agency for Healthcare Research and Quality (AHRQ)
13. http://www.guidelines.gov
14. *Healthy People 2010*
15. outcomes research

Acquiring Knowledge in Nursing

1. You could have identified any of the following ways of acquiring knowledge in nursing. Some possible examples of each way of acquiring nursing knowledge are provided.
    a. Tradition: giving a report on hospitalized patients in a specific way or organizing the care provided to the patients in a specific, structured way
    b. Authority: expert nurses, educators, and authors of articles or books
    c. Borrowing: using knowledge from medicine or psychology in nursing practice
    d. Trial and error: positioning a patient to reduce his or her discomfort during an intramuscular injection or trying different interventions to help patients sleep at night
    e. Personal experience: obtaining knowledge by being in a clinical agency and providing care to patients and families
    f. Role-modeling: a new graduate in an internship being mentored by an expert nurse who models excellent clinical behavior
    g. Intuition: knowing that a patient's condition is deteriorating but having no concrete data to support this feeling or hunch
    h. Reasoning: reasoning from the general to the specific or deductive reasoning; reasoning from the specific to the general or inductive reasoning
    i. Research: quantitative, qualitative, and outcomes research methods
2. personal experience

3. a. novice
    b. advanced beginner
    c. competent
    d. proficient
    e. expert
4. research, empirical, or scientific
5. intuition
6. traditions
7. deductive reasoning
8. Important outcomes focused on: (a) patient health status (signs, symptoms, functional status, morbidity, mortality), (b) patient satisfaction, (c) costs related to health care, (d) quality of care, (e) quality of care provider, (f) provider satisfaction, and (g) access to care by patients and families.

Making Connections

Linking Research Methods to Types of Research
1. b
2. b
3. a
4. b
5. a
6. a
7. a
8. b

Determining the Strength of Levels of Research Evidence
Rank order of the levels of research evidence is: 4, 1, 3, 2, 6, 5

Nurses' Role in Research
1. a
2. e
3. a and/or b
4. d and/or e
5. c
6. b and/or c
7. d
8. c
9. e
10. d & e

Exercises in Critical Appraisal

Research Methods
1. c
2. c
3. b

Researchers' Credentials
1. Bindler, Massey, Shultz, Mills, and Short all have PhDs, which is a research educational preparation. Bindler also is a registered nurse (RN) who is certified (C) in an area of specialization, supporting her clinical expertise. Massey is a registered dietitian (RD), which is a clinical strength with the nutritional focus of this study. The study was supported by the Society for Pediatric Nurses, Delta Chi Chapter of Sigma Theta Tau International, and Washington State University. These individuals were employed by Washington State University and most faculty members are involved with research. These authors have the educational, research, and clinical expertise to conduct this study.
2. Padula is PhD-prepared, which is a research degree, and employed by the College of Nursing, University of Rhode Island. She is also a certified specialist (CS), indicating clinical expertise. Yeaw has a PhD and is employed in the College of Pharmacy in the same university indicating her educational expertise. Both Padula and Yeaw are registered nurses (RN), indicating clinical expertise in nursing. Both of these researchers had conducted a previous study in this area that is cited in the reference list of the article. Mistry has a master's degree and is also working in the College of Nursing. These researchers received a grant from the National Institute of Nursing Research and support from the College of Nursing at the University of Rhode Island. Thus these authors have the educational, research, and clinical expertise to conduct this study. This information was available in the research article.

3. Schachman is doctorally (PhD) prepared and an associate professor at Montana State University, Bozeman, Montana. Her educational preparation (PhD) and position as an associate professor indicate that she has been actively involved in conducting research. *Nursing Research* is a prestigious research journal for nurses to publish their studies. Dr. Schachman's credentials identify her as a certified advanced-practice nurse (APRN-BC), which documents her clinical expertise. She has developed programs to assist new military moms adapt. Dr. Schachman is married to a man who just retired from the Marine Corps after 25 years of military service. Thus this author has the research, educational, and clinical expertise, as well as personal experience, to conduct this study. This information was obtained by reviewing the author information at the bottom of the first page of the article and by Googling "Schachman, Kathleen."

Going Beyond

Critical Appraisal of Study Title and Abstract
Title: Padula et al. (2009) entitled their study "A home-based nurse-coached inspiratory muscle training intervention in heart failure." This title clearly identifies the study population as patients with heart failure and indicates the type of study, quasi-experimental quantitative study. The intervention for the study is clearly identified but not the outcome or dependent variables. The study identifies an interesting intervention that patients might use to improve their heart failure condition.

Abstract: Critical Appraisal of the abstract for the Bindler et al. (2007) study indicated that the study problem was clearly identified and significant. The study purpose and the key findings from the study were also concisely presented. The abstract was very brief and would have been strengthened by identification of the study design, sample size and framework.

CHAPTER 2—INTRODUCTION TO THE QUANTITATIVE RESEARCH PROCESS

Key Terms
1. m
2. s
3. a
4. d
5. r
6. c
7. i
8. l
9. q
10. t
11. n
12. o
13. f
14. k
15. h
16. g
17. e
18. j
19. p
20. b

Key Ideas

Control in Quantitative Research
1. highly controlled
2. quasi-experimental and experimental
3. descriptive and correlational
4. experimental
5. nonrandom or nonprobability, random or probability
6. natural
7. highly controlled
8. experimental
9. partially controlled

Steps of the Research Process
1. problem-solving and nursing processes
2. Step 1: Research problem and purpose
   Step 2: Literature review

Step 3: Study framework
Step 4: Research objectives, questions, or hypotheses
Step 5: Study variables
Step 6: Assumptions
Step 7: Limitations
Step 8: Research design
Step 9: Population and sample
Step 10: Methods of measurement
Step 11: Data collection
Step 12: Data analysis
Step 13: Research outcomes; and you might have also included the answers communication of findings and use of findings in practice

3. Assumptions are statements taken for granted or considered true, even though they have not been scientifically tested.

4. You could identify any of the following assumptions or other assumptions you have noted in a research report.
   a. People want to assume control of their own health problems.
   b. Stress should be avoided.
   c. Health is a priority for most people.
   d. People in underserved areas feel underserved.
   e. Attitudes can be measured with a scale.
   f. Most measurable attitudes are held strongly enough to direct behavior.
   g. Health professionals view health care in a manner different from that of laypersons.
   h. Human biological and chemical factors show less variation than do cultural and socialfactors.
   i. People operate on the basis of cognitive information.
   j. Increased knowledge about an event lowers anxiety about the event.
   k. Receipt of health care at home is preferable to receipt of care in an institution.

5. theoretical and methodological

6. Answer can include methodological or theoretical limitations. The methodological limitations include such factors as nonrepresentative sample, small sample size, weak design, single setting, instruments with limited reliability and validity, limited control over data collection, weak implementation of the treatment, and improper use of statistical analyses. Theoretical limitations include weak definitions of concepts in the framework, weak conceptual definitions of variables, poorly developed study framework, and unclear links between study variables and framework concepts.

7. A pilot study is a smaller version of a proposed study that is conducted to develop and/or refine the study methodology, such as the treatment, measurement instruments, or data collection process to be used in the larger study.

8. You could identify any of the following reasons for conducting a pilot study:
   a. To determine whether the proposed study is feasible (e.g., Are the subjects available? Does the researcher have the time and money to conduct the study?).
   b. To develop or refine a research treatment or intervention.
   c. To develop a protocol for the implementation of a treatment.
   d. To identify problems with the design.
   e. To determine whether the sample is representative of the population or whether the sampling technique is effective.
   f. To examine the reliability and validity of the research instruments.
   g. To develop or refine data collection instruments.
   h. To refine the data collection and analysis plan.
   i. To give the researcher experience with the subjects, setting, methodology, and methods of measurement.
   j. To try out data analysis techniques.

Reading Research Reports

1. You could identify any three of the following research journals.
   a. *Advances in Nursing Science*

   b. *Applied Nursing Research*
   c. *Biological Research for Nursing*
   d. *Clinical Nursing Research: An International Journal*
   e. *Journal of Nursing Scholarship*
   f. *International Journal of Nursing Studies*
   g. *Nursing Research*
   h. *Nursing Science Quarterly*
   i. *Qualitative Nursing Research*
   j. *Research in Nursing & Health*
   k. *Scholarly Inquiry for Nursing Practice: An International Journal*
   l. *Western Journal of Nursing Research*
2. Look in clinical journals and see which ones have several research articles in each issue. You could identify any two of the following journals:
   a. *Issues in Comprehensive Pediatric Nursing*
   b. *Journal of Transcultural Nursing*
   c. *Heart & Lung: Journal of Acute and Critical Care*
   d. *Journal of Nursing Education*
   e. *Birth*
   f. *Nursing Diagnosis*
   g. *Public Health Nursing*
   h. *The Diabetes Educator*
   i. *Maternal-Child Nursing Journal*
   j. *Journal of Nursing Education*
   k. *Journal of Pediatric Nursing*
   l. *Archives of Psychiatric Nursing*
3. introduction, methods, results, and discussion
4. design, sample, setting, methods of measurement, and data collection process. The methods section also includes the treatment if that is applicable to the type of study being conducted, such as for quasi-experimental and experimental studies.
5. major findings, limitations of the study, conclusions drawn from the findings, implications of the findings for nursing, and recommendations for further research
6. introduction section
7. theories and studies
8. skimming, comprehending, and analyzing
9. comprehending step involves identifying the steps of the research process.
10. analyzing step involves determining the value of the research report's content by examining the quality and completeness of the steps of the research process and the links among these steps

Making Connections

Types of Quantitative Research

1.	c	11.	b
2.	a	12.	a
3.	b	13.	c
4.	a	14.	a
5.	c	15.	c
6.	d	16.	a
7.	a	17.	b
8.	b	18.	a
9.	c	19.	a
10.	d	20.	b

Crossword Puzzle

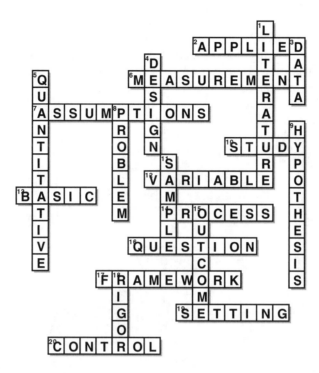

Exercises in Critical Appraisal

Type of Quantitative Research
1. b
2. c
3. e

Type of Setting
4. b   Bindler et al. (2007) study was conducted in a partially controlled setting: Data were collected in large rooms at the schools and the rooms were separated into stations for testing of the different study variables.
5. a   Padula et al. (2009) study was conducted in a natural setting: Research assistants made home visits to implement the treatment and to collect the data for the dependent variables.
6. a   Schachman (2010) study was conducted in a natural setting: The researcher conducted the study interviews in the fathers' homes.

Type of Research Conducted (Applied or Basic)
7. a
8. a
9. a

CHAPTER 3—INTRODUCTION TO THE QUALITATIVE RESEARCH PROCESS

Key Terms and Persons

1.	d	9.	f	17.	b
2.	c	10.	e	18.	f
3.	j	11.	m	19.	d
4.	k	12.	i	20.	a
5.	n	13.	g	21.	e
6.	o	14.	a	22.	c
7.	p	15.	h		
8.	b	16.	l		

23. Gathering data first-hand by being present in a situation.
24. Labeling words and phrases on the transcript of an interview or focus group that indicates a more abstract meaning; codes are synthesized and may lead to themes in the data.
25. Study of the past that provides nurses increased understanding of the profession.
26. Open and honest communication between the researcher and participant that is a critical element in qualitative research and shapes the collection, analysis, and interpretation of the data.

Key Ideas
1. value laden or subjective
2. individual or person
3. reality, beliefs
4. immersed
5. native
6. unstructured
7. moderator or facilitator
8. field notes
9. snowball or network
10. phenomenology
11. Heidegger
12. sociology
13. case study
14. ethnography
15. first-hand
16. nonprobability
17. interviews
18. organize, code, retrieve
19. Culture
20. historical research

Making Connections

Comparing Qualitative and Quantitative Research Methodologies

1. QN
2. QL
3. QN
4. QN
5. QL
6. QL
7. QL
8. QN
9. QN
10. QN

Approaches to Qualitative Research

1. E
2. G
3. E
4. P
5. E
6. H
7. P
8. G
9. H
10. G

Crossword Puzzle

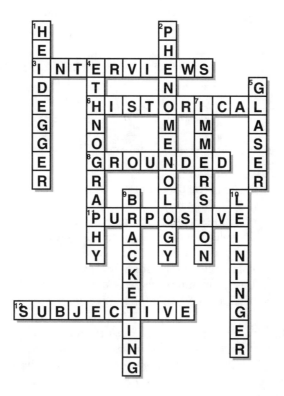

Exercises in Critical Appraisal

1. "Explore the lived experience of first-time fatherhood from the unique perspective of military men who are deployed to combat regions during birth" (p. 225).

2. Phenomenology was used because the "focus is on the lived experience from the perspective of the informants and because little is known about this experience" (p. 226).

3. Participants were recruited during a briefing held in Okinawa after deployment in the Middle East. The men were self-identified as first-time fathers and the researcher invited them to participate. Purposive sampling was used.

4. "...an open-ended interview was conducted by the researcher at the father's home. Each man was asked a single question: 'What is it like to become a father while deployed overseas to a combat region?' Follow-up questions were used only as required for clarification. All interviews lasted from 40 to 65 minutes and were audiotaped. Following each interview, field notes were recorded to document observations about the father and the environment. Audiotaped interviews and field notes were transcribed verbatim within 72 hours" (p. 226).

5. Extensive journal writing about one's own perspectives on the research topic and being mentored by a peer researcher who was not familiar with the topic and can provide a potentially less biased view of the research topic.

6. Table

Main Theme I: Disruption of the Protector and Provider Role	Main Theme II: Restoration of the Protector and Provider Role
Worry: A traumatic and lonely childbirth	Communication: The ties that bind
Lost opportunity	
Guilt: An absent father	
Fear of death and dismemberment	

7. Answers will vary according to the student.
8. "Although the first-time fathers who participated in this study reflected the diversity of the military in terms of ethnicity, age, and education, each of the men belonged to a traditional nuclear family. This study was not focused on different kinds of families, despite the many family types that exist. In addition, the experiences of these new fathers are examined within an ethnocentric view of fatherhood common in Western countries; all new and expectant fathers may not hold the same expectations of their role. The results cannot be generalized beyond the participants in this study because lived experiences differ for individuals according to context and time… Lastly, the interviews were conducted 2 to 6 months after the children were born; thus the possibility exists that the recall of events and feelings were diminished through time delay" (pp. 229-230).
9. Impact of doula care on the deployed fathers has not been examined.
10. Relevance of the findings is that nurses have an increased understanding of new fathers' experiences and perspectives and can assist and support these men involved in the fatherhood role. "This information can be used to set the stage for healthy reunions, which may take place at military bases and within communities across the globe, and thus is of benefit to all nurses working with military families" (p. 230).

CHAPTER 4—EXAMINING ETHICS IN NURSING RESEARCH

Key Terms
1. g
2. a
3. i
4. k
5. j
6. e
7. m
8. c
9. o
10. f
11. d
12. n
13. h
14. b
15. l

Key Ideas
1. a. Disclosure of essential study information to the subject
    b. Comprehension of this information by the subject
    c. Competency of the subject to give consent
    d. Voluntary consent by the subject to participate in the study
2. Essential information in a study consent form:
    a. Introduction of the research activities
    b. Statement of the research purpose
    c. Explanation of study procedures
    d. Description of risks for discomfort and harm
    e. Description of benefits
    f. Disclosure of alternatives
    g. Assurance of anonymity and confidentiality

    h.   Offer to answer questions
    i.   Option to withdraw
    j.   Contact information for the researcher(s)
3. Voluntary
4. Diminished autonomy
5. Institutional Review Board (IRB)
6. a.   Exempt from review
    b.   Expedited review
    c.   Complete or full review
7. To determine the benefit-risk ratio, you need to assess the benefits and risks of the sampling method, consent process, procedures, and outcomes of the study. The proposed study needs to indicate that informed consent and Health Insurance Portability and Accountability Act (HIPAA) release will be obtained from the subjects and selection and treatment of the subjects during the study will be fair. The type of knowledge generated from the study also needs to be examined to determine how this knowledge will impact the subjects (therapeutic or nontherapeutic) and influence nursing practice. The risks need to be reduced, if possible, and should not cause serious harm to the subjects. The benefits need to be maximized, if possible. If the benefits adequately outweigh the risks for the study, then the benefit-risk ratio usually indicates that the study is ethical to conduct.
8. Exempt from review is the most likely answer, but the type of review is determined by the IRB of the agency where the study is to be conducted.
9. Complete review
10. Possible answers include:
    a.   Fabrication of data in the research report
    b.   Falsification of data in the research report
    c.   Forging of data
    d.   Manipulation of the design or methods of a study to obtain the results desired
    e.   Selectively retaining or manipulating study data
    f.   Manipulation of data analyses to obtain the results desired
    g.   Plagiarism of another author and/or researcher's work
    h.   Included as an author on a publication when the person did not have direct involvement in the conduct of a study
11. Office of Scientific Integrity Review (OSIR) and Office of Scientific Integrity (OSI)
12. Yes, this is an area of concern in nursing. Articles have been written by nurses and published in nursing journals outlining the concerns and actions to be taken to control research misconduct in the discipline. Journal editors have expressed concerns about research misconduct and have developed guidelines for managing such problems. None of the major misconduct problems mentioned in the text had nurses as principal investigators but sometimes nurses have been on research teams that experienced incidences of research misconduct.
13. Yes. An increasing number of animals are being used by nurse scientists to generate basic research knowledge for the profession. Most of the animals used in research are mice and rats.
14. American Association for Accreditation of Laboratory Animal Care (AAALAC)
15. Best answer is yes. Rationale might focus on the importance of animal studies to generate basic knowledge to provide a basis for conducting applied studies on humans. Agencies exist to protect the animals and ensure humane treatment during research.

    If you answered no, your rationale might focus on the inhumane aspects of using animals in studies or the cost of using animals in research.

Making Connections

Historical Events, Ethical Codes, and Regulations

1.	b	6.	a
2.	c	7.	d
3.	d	8.	b
4.	b	9.	a
5.	c	10.	c

Ethical Principles

1. c
2. a
3. c

4. b
5. b or c

Federal Regulations Influencing the Conduct of Research

1. a
2. c
3. a

4. b
5. c

Ethics of Published Studies

1. d
2. a
3. b

4. e
5. c

Crossword Puzzle

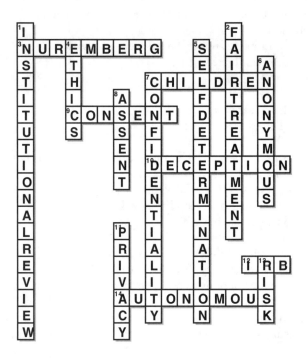

Exercises in Critical Appraisal

1. Bindler, Massey, Shultz, Mills, and Short's (2007) study appeared to be ethical as indicated by the following excerpt from their research article. The researchers received Institutional Review Board (IRB) approvals: "The protocol was approved by the Institutional Review Boards of Spokane, Washington, and Washington State University, and the school board of the district where the study was conducted" (p. 205). The researchers obtained consent from the parents and assent from the children to participate in their study and the study information was provided in both English and Spanish languages to ensure communication with the parents. "If they signed a consent, their children were informed about the study and could choose whether to sign an assent and participate" (Bindler et al., 2007, p. 205) (informed consent process). This study appears to be ethical, because the risks are minimal and the benefits are strong, resulting in a positive benefit-risk ratio. However, the ethics of the study would have been stronger if the researchers would have mentioned HIPAA information.

2. Padula, Yeaw, and Mistry's (2009) study appeared to be ethical. The researchers indicated that if the subjects met eligibility criteria then informed consent was obtained from them. The study would have been stronger if the researchers would have provided a little more detail about the informed consent process. The subjects were treated fairly because they were randomly assigned to either the treatment group or comparison

group. The researchers detailed their IRB approval in the following excerpt: "This study was reviewed and approved by three institutional review boards. Recruiting physicians signed the Federal Wide Assurance forms [HIPAA], and RAs (research assistants) completed human subjects' certifications" (Padula et al., 2009, p. 219). This study has potential therapeutic benefits for the patients with heart failure in the treatment group and involves minimal risks. Thus the study has a positive benefit-risk ratio

3. Schachman's (2010) study documented the institutional review and informed consent processes in the following excerpt but did not include a discussion of HIPAA. "Approval from the university's institutional review board was granted prior to the study. After obtaining informed consent from each father, an open-ended interview was conducted by the researcher at the father's home" (Schachman, 2010, p. 226). This study provided nurses with a better understanding of the needs of first-time fathers who are combat-deployed during the births of their infants. Additional, ideas were identified to better prepare and support these men in their fatherhood role. This study has minimal, if any, risks and several potential benefits for expanding the knowledge of nurses in providing care to fathers in the military.

CHAPTER 5—RESEARCH PROBLEMS, PURPOSES, AND HYPOTHESES

Key Terms

Chapter Terms

1. d
2. i
3. h
4. g
5. j
6. k
7. f
8. e
9. a
10. c
11. b

Types of Hypotheses

1. h
2. g
3. b
4. e
5. c
6. a
7. d
8. f

Variables and Key Terms

1. a
2. d
3. f
4. c
5. e
6. b

Key Ideas

Research Problem and Purpose
1. variables for quantitative and outcomes studies and concepts for qualitative studies, population, and setting
2. a. has an impact on or is used to guide nursing practice
   b. builds on previous research
   c. promotes theory testing and development
   d. addresses current concerns or priorities in nursing
3. You might have identified any of the following agencies or organizations: National Institute for Nursing Research (NINR), American Association of Critical-Care Nurses (AACN), American Association of Occupational Health Nurses (AAOHN), Oncology Nursing Society (ONS), American Organization of Nurse Executives (AONE), or Agency for Healthcare Research and Quality (AHRQ). You might have identified other nursing and health care professional organizations that have research priorities identified.
4. a. researchers' expertise
   b. financial commitment
   c. availability of subjects, facility, and equipment
   d. study's ethical considerations
5. educational, research or clinical expertise

Exercises in Critical Appraisal

Bindler, Massey, Shultz, Mills, and Short (2007) Study

1. a. Significance of the problem: "One in four Americans is at risk for developing metabolic syndrome (Ford, Giles, & Diets, 2002; Roberts, Dunn, Jean, & Lardinois, 2000). Life-style, environment, and genetic component are influential in the syndrome… Due to an epidemic in youth obesity and sedentary behaviors, there is an increasing need to describe the factors associated with the development of insulin resistance in youths" (Bindler et al., 2007, p. 202).

    b. Background of the problem: "Metabolic syndrome, also known as dysmetabolic syndrome, syndrome X, or insulin resistance syndrome, is characterized by a group of risk factors and is often a precursor to both diabetes and cardiovascular disease. These risk factors cluster in individuals and populations, both in adults and in youths… These criteria reflect the major metabolic components of the syndrome, which are abdominal obesity, atherogenic dyslipidemia, increased blood pressure (BP), insulin resistance, proinflammatory state, and prothrombotic state (Grundy, Brewer, Cleeman, Smith, & Lenfant, 2004). Other groups have recommended somewhat different criteria, leading to confusion among clinicians (See Table 1 for a summary of adult criteria recommendations for metabolic syndrome) (Zimmet, Magliano, Matsuzawa, Alberti, & Shaw, 2005)" Bindler et al., 2007, p. 201).

    c. Problem statement: "Children in general, and those from Native American and Hispanic groups, in particular, are underrepresented in diabetes and cardiovascular disease origins research. There is scant application of identification methods for metabolic syndrome in the nursing literature. More information is needed to establish the contribution of various characteristics to insulin resistance in children, and translational research is needed so that findings can be applied by nurses and other health professionals in pediatric settings. Descriptive data about children, particular from disparate ethnic groups, will help to identify children at highest risk so that appropriate interventions can be identified. Clear guidelines for nurses will assist in applying findings about metabolic syndrome to pediatric settings with youths" (Bindler et al., 2007, p. 204). This study includes several problem statements that clearly indicate what is not known and provide a basis for this study.

2. Study purpose: "The purpose of this study was to describe serum insulin levels and to investigate their relationships to metabolic syndrome criteria in a multiethnic sample of school children" (Bindler et al., 2007, p. 204).

3. The problem and purpose are significant because of the increasing number of obese, sedentary school-age children who are at risk for developing metabolic syndrome. For those developing this insulin resistance syndrome, research has documented that they are at increased risk for diabetes and cardiovascular disease. Because metabolic syndrome is caused by life-style choices of diet and exercise activities that can be altered, it is important to identify the children at risk and to provide appropriate interventions. Care of children requires a unique knowledge base for nurses to provide interventions to promote health and prevent illness, such as metabolic syndrome. In addition, identifying and treating children with metabolic syndrome can greatly improve their future health and decrease health care costs.

4. Yes, the variables, population, and settings are identified.

    a. This is a predictive correlational study. The dependent variable of insulin level was predicted using the independent variables metabolic syndrome, gender, age, race, BMI percentile, glucose, triglycerides, HDL-C, systolic blood pressure, and diastolic blood pressure.

    b. Population: School-age children attending fourth to eighth grades

    c. Settings: Public elementary and middle schools in a predominately agricultural area of central Washington State

5. The problem and purpose are feasible because (1) the study was funded by a Sigma Theta Tau Chapter and Washington State University College of Nursing; (2) Bindler had previous research in this area and clinical expertise and the other researchers had educational and clinical expertise to conduct this study, as discussed in Chapter 2 of this Study Guide; (3) adequate subjects were available to participate in the study because the population was school-age children and the settings were public elementary and middle schools; (4) school personnel were supportive of the study; (5) arrangements were made to obtain the blood samples needed for the study and to conduct the laboratory analysis of the serum; and (5) the study was ethical and protected the rights of the subjects.

Padula, Yeaw, and Mistry (2009) Study

1. a. Significance of the problem: "Heart failure (HF) is a major public health problem affecting more than 5 million people in the United States and is the leading cause of repeat hospitalizations (American Heart Association, 2000). People with HF are living longer but with disabling symptoms, particularly dyspnea, that erode quality of life (QOL)… Decreased strength of inspiratory muscles (IMs) may contribute to the dyspnea in HF (Vibarel et al., 2002)" (p. 217).

    b. Background of the problem: "Inspiratory muscle training (IMT) has been shown to increase the performance of the IMs in patients with chronic obstructive pulmonary disease (COPD) (Larson, Covey, & Corbridge, 2002). COPD and chronic HF are diseases with similar muscular problems, including the mechanisms and clinical impact of muscle dysfunction (Caroci & Lareau, 2004)" (p. 217).

    c. Problem statement: "Further research is needed to clearly specify dosing and to determine the impact of IMT on dyspnea and QOL. All of the studies were atheoretical; one RCT (randomized controlled trial) (Dall'Ago et al., 2006) was home-based and was conducted by a physical therapist. This research expands and extends previous research using nurse-coached IMT intervention in the home and based on Self-Efficacy Theory" (p. 218).

2. The purpose of this study was to determine the effects of a 3-month nurse-coached IMT program on inspiratory muscle strength (IMS), dyspnea, self-efficacy for breathing, and health-related QOL (HRQOL) outcomes for patients with HF. The purpose in this study lacked completeness and was restated to include the independent variable (IMT) and all the dependent variables.

3. The problem and purpose are significant because over 5 million people have HF in the U.S. HF has high morbidity and mortality rates for those afflicted with this chronic disease. HF results in disabling symptoms and repeat hospitalizations for patients, requiring billions of health care dollars to manage this condition.

4. The variables, population, and setting are clearly identified in this study.

    a. Variables: This is a quasi-experimental study that included the independent variable (treatment) of nurse-coached IMT program. The dependent or outcome variables included inspiratory muscle strength (IMS), dyspnea, self-efficacy related to breathing, and physical/functional and psychosocial dimensions of HRQOL.

    b. Population for the study was adults with HF.

    c. Setting for the study was subjects' homes.

5. This study was feasible because of the expertise of the researchers, the external national funding for the study, access to the subjects and equipment needed to conduct the study, and the ethical nature of the study. Padula and Yeaw have strong educational preparation (PhD) to conduct this study and have published previous research in this area. Padula and Yeaw have nursing clinical expertise and Mistry has pharmacology expertise. The authors had access to several adults with HF by recruiting from physicians' offices, home-care agencies, provider referral, and newspaper advertisement. This study was funded by the National Institute of Nursing Research (NINR) and graduate assistant support was provided by the College of Nursing, University of Rhode Island. The study was ethical because the authors received institutional review board (IRB) approval from the appropriate agencies and informed consent was obtained from the subjects.

Schachman (2010) study

1. a. Significance and background of the problem: "Over the past three decades, men have become a virtually universal presence in the delivery room. Birth attendance by fathers is a culturally prescribed expectation in the United States (Knoester, Petts, & Eggebeen, 2007; Lamb, 2003). The father's presence during childbirth is thought to impact not only maternal outcomes such as the labor process and satisfaction (Essex & Pickett, 2008; Hodnett, Gates, Hofmeyer, & Sakala, 2007) but also family well-being and the development of a favorable father-child relationship (Pleck & Masciadrelli, 2004; Premberg, Hellstrom, & Berg, 2008). Today, over 90% of fathers in the United States attend the birth of their children… An exception to this, however, is men in the military who are separated geographically from their laboring partners, due to combat deployment. Over 100,000 service members are deployed currently in combat regions; more than half of them are married and below the age of 30 years (Department of Defense, Statistical Information Analysis Division, 2009)" (p. 225).

    b. Problem statement: "Although important insight into the father's perspectives of childbirth has been demonstrated, the perspective of men who are absent during this important event remains unknown… Better understanding of new fatherhood in this population may form more helpful and supportive approaches to facilitate fathers' participation in the new role, despite the challenges of a stressful combat environment and geographic separation" (Schachman, 2010, p. 226).

2. "The purpose of this qualitative study was to explore the lived experience of first-time fatherhood from the unique perspective of military men who are deployed to combat regions during birth" (Schachman, 2010, p. 226).

3. The problem is significant because the research has identified the benefits of having fathers in the labor room and fathers combat-deployed cannot participate in the birth of their children. Many men are currently deployed to combat regions and this number is growing each year. More than half of the men are married and less than 30 years of age. Thus they are more likely to become fathers during their military service. In addition, the problem statement clearly indicates the gap in the knowledge base and the need to understand these combat-deployed fathers' perspective about being absent during this important event. The purpose builds upon the problem statement and clearly indicates the focus of the study.

4. This study clearly identified the research concept, population, and type of study to be conducted but the setting is unclear.
   a. The research concept is lived experience of first-time fatherhood and the type of study is qualitative.
   b. The population is first-time fathers who are combat-deployed.
   c. The setting is not clear in the purpose but is clearly identified in the abstract as a military base in Okinawa, Japan.

5. The study was feasible because the researcher was able to access the 17 subjects that were needed for the study from a military base in Japan. The study was conducted by a PhD-prepared certified advanced-practice nurse who is an associate professor at Montana State University. This information about the author indicates she has the research, educational, and clinical expertise to conduct this study. The study requires limited supplies for copying, taping interviews, and typing the data for analysis, and it requires no equipment. The study is ethical, and institutional board review was conducted by appropriate agencies and informed consent was obtained from the subjects who participated in the study.

Making Connections

Objectives, Questions, and Hypotheses

1. b, c, d, g
2. a, c, e, g
3. b, c, e, f
4. a, d, g, h
5. b, d, g, h
6. b, c, d, g
7. a, c, d, g
8. b, c, e, f
9. a, c, e, g
10. b, d, g, h
11. Increased age, decreased family support, and decreased health status are related to decreased self-care abilities in nursing home residents.
12. Low-back massage is no more effective in decreasing perceptions of low-back pain than no massage in patients with chronic low-back pain.
13. Nurses' perceived work stress, internal locus of control, and social support are not related to their psychological symptoms.

Exercises in Critical Appraisal

Bindler et al. (2007) Study

1. Bindler et al. (p. 204) stated research questions to guide their study: "1. What are the fasting serum insulin levels in a multiethnic sample of school children in central Washington State? 2. What are the relationships between insulin levels and the criteria for metabolic syndrome in a multiethnic sample of children in central Washington State? 3. What are the relationships between reported dietary intake and metabolic syndrome criteria? 4. Which data predict insulin levels in this multiethnic sample of children? 5. How can the information learned in this study be used by pediatric nurses in clinical settings?"

2. The research questions are clearly stated and direct the development of the design, the data analysis, and interpretation of the findings. This is a correlational study with a descriptive, predictive correlational design. The first research question focuses on description of insulin levels in children, questions 2 and 3 focus on examining relationships among study variables, and question 4 focuses on prediction of insulin levels. Question 5 is not linked to the study design and might have been omitted. The link to practice or "Clinical Implications" are best included in the Discussion section and do need a research question. The "Results" section clearly identifies the research questions and descriptive analyses are conducted to address question 1, correlational analyses for questions 2 and 3, and regression analysis is conducted to address question 4. Question 5 is addressed in the Discussion section.

Padula et al. (2009) Study
1. This study had aims or objectives, a research question, and a hypothesis. "Primary aim was to determine the effect of 3 months of nurse-coached IMT with respect to IM strength and perceived dyspnea. The secondary aims were to determine the effect of IMT with respect to self-efficacy for breathing and physical/functional and psychosocial dimensions of HRQOL. The research question is as follows: Is a home-based IMT intervention more effective in improving IM strength, dyspnea, self-efficacy for breathing, and HRQOL outcomes than an educational comparison group?" (p. 219). "It was hypothesized that IMT would increase the strength of IMs, decrease dyspnea, and have a positive effect on health-related QOL (HRQOL)" (p. 217).
2. Hypothesis is best developed to direct the conduct of this study, because it is a quasi-experimental study conducted to determine the effect of IMT (independent variable) on selected dependent or outcome variables. It is confusing to the reader to include aims (objectives), research question, and hypothesis. The aims and research question seem to be repetitive and do not provide complete, clear direction to the study. However, the hypothesis is the most complete and clearly stated to direct the study and the most appropriate for this type of study. The data analyses in the Results section of this article do not clearly link to the aims, research question, or hypothesis. The Results section is organized by the study dependent variables instead of the study hypothesis.

Schachman (2010) Study
1. This is a qualitative study that has no objectives, questions, or hypotheses. The research purpose provides direction for this study, and this is common in qualitative studies.
2. No objectives, questions, or hypotheses

Making Connections

Understanding Study Variables
1. a
2. b
3. c
4. a
5. b
6. b
7. b
8. c
9. a
10. c
11. c
12. b
13. a
14. b
15. a

Exercises in Critical Appraisal

Bindler et al. (2007) Study

1. Study variables

Variables	Type of Variable
Gender	Independent variable
Age	Independent variable
Race	Independent variable
Body mass index (BMI) percentile	Independent variable
Glucose	Independent variable
Triglycerides	Independent variable
HDL Cholesterol	Independent variable
Systolic and diastolic blood pressure	Independent variable
Fasting serum insulin level	Dependent variable

2. Conceptual and Operational Definitions for Fasting Serum Insulin Levels
    a. Conceptual definition: Serum insulin level is a physiological indicator of metabolic functioning and health status and high insulin levels have been linked to metabolic syndrome or insulin resistance.
    b. Operational definition: Fasting serum insulin levels were obtained from blood draws "completed in the early morning by the licensed phlebotomist after the children had fasted for at least 10 hours" (Bindler et al., 2007, p. 205).
3. The conceptual and operational definitions for serum insulin levels are clearly expressed in the study. The conceptual definition provides a strong link to the operational definition, which is exceptionally strong and appropriate for this study. However, the study lacks a clearly identified framework so the conceptual definition lacks a theoretical basis.
4. Demographic variables included in this study were: gender, age, family history (cardiovascular disease, diabetes, overweight, and smoking), and smoking history (see Table 3, p. 207). Age and gender were also used as independent variables in the regression analysis (see Table 8, p. 211).

Padula et al. (2009) Study

1. Study Variables

Variables	Type of Variable
IMT	Independent variable
IMS	Dependent variable
Dyspnea	Dependent variable
Self-efficacy related to breathing	Dependent variable
Physical/functional and psychosocial HRQOL	Dependent variable
Clinical assessment (weight, BP, pulse, respiratory rate, respiratory pattern, edema, lung sounds)	Dependent variables

2. Conceptual and Operational Definitions for IMT Intervention
    Conceptual definition: "Bandura's Self-Efficacy Theory guided the intervention for the experimental group (IMT)… Vicarious experiences for the IMT group were accomplished by observing the demonstration of the tack of using the Threshold Device, thus 'modeling' the instruction and demonstration provided by the RA. Performance accomplishment was achieved by 'mastering' the technique of inspiring into the device with a nose clip in place… thus providing tangible evidence of progress" (Padula et al., 2009, p. 220).

Operational definition: "The Threshold Device (Healthscan) was used for resistive IMT breathing training... Training consisted of demonstration by the RAs, with return demonstration at baseline followed by a week of device use" (Padula et al., 2009, p. 219).

3. The researchers provide very clear and appropriate conceptual and operational definitions for the IMT intervention in this study. The conceptual definition is clearly linked to the study framework, Bandura's Self-Efficacy Theory. The implementation of the IMT study intervention is clearly described in the operational definition.

4. The demographic variables in this study include: gender, marital status, age in years, and New York Heart Association (NYHA) classification (see Table 1 [p. 221] in the article and the Sample description in the Results section).

Schachman (2010) Study

1. Research concept: lived experience of first-time fatherhood

2. Conceptual definition: This phenomenological study was conducted to conceptually define the lived experience of first-time fatherhood in combat-deployed troops. In the study, "Five theme clusters emerged that were subsumed under two main themes of *disruption of protector and provider role*, and *restoration of the protector and provider role*. The essence of the experience of first-time fatherhood in men deployed to combat regions is captured in these two main themes" (Schachman, 2010, p. 227). These themes are detailed in the article in Appendix B.

3. The conceptual definition was extremely strong, supported by the data that were included in this article, and relevant data were presented in Table 2 (p. 227) and in the narrative of the article.

4. The demographic variables for this study included: duration of combat deployment, marital status, educational level, age, and ethnicity.

CHAPTER 6—UNDERSTANDING THE LITERATURE REVIEW IN PUBLISHED STUDIES

Key Terms

1. q
2. k
3. e
4. s
5. i
6. o
7. r
8. l
9. j
10. d

11. p
12. t
13. b
14. c
15. h
16. a
17. m
18. f
19. g
20. n

Key Ideas

1. theoretical and empirical sources
2. compare and combine findings from the study with the literature to determine current knowledge of a phenomenon
3. ethnographic and quantitative research (descriptive, correlational, quasi-experimental, and experimental studies)
4. historical research
5. landmark
6. known and not known
7. published 5 years before publication of the report
8. secondary source
9. electronic databases
10. Internet
11. a. selecting databases to search
    b. selecting keywords to use
    c. storing references by using reference management software
    d. locating relevant literature

12. Cumulative Index to Nursing & Allied Health Literature (CINAHL)
13. thesaurus
14. store information retrieved from computer reference databases
15. *Annual Review of Nursing Research*
16. synthesis
17. introduction, empirical literature, theoretical literature, and summary
18. Key terms based on this study title to direct the literature review include: spirituality, family, resuscitation, support, psychosocial, adults.
19. a. An integrative review of literature is a review conducted to identify, analyze, and synthesize the results from independent studies to determine the current knowledge in a particular area.
    b. A meta-analysis includes performing statistical analyses to integrate and synthesize findings of completed studies to determine what is known and not known about a particular research area.
20. a. the names of databases used
    b. the date the search is performed
    c. the exact search strategy that is used
    d. the number of articles that are found
    e. the percentage of relevant articles that are found

Making Connections

Theoretical and Empirical Sources

1.	T	7.	E
2.	E	8.	E
3.	E	9.	T
4.	T	10.	T
5.	T	11.	E
6.	E	12.	T

Primary and Secondary Sources

1.	S	6.	P
2.	P	7.	P
3.	P	8.	S
4.	S	9.	P
5.	S	10.	P

The Purpose of the Literature Review in Quantitative Research Methodologies
Correct answers include any four of the following:
    a. summarize the background and significance of the research problem
    b. document what is known and not known about the problem
    c. describe the theoretical framework
    d. justify the methods used in the study
    e. compare the results of the study with results of previous studies
    f. synthesize the current results with previous results

The Literature in Qualitative Research Methods
1. d
2. c
3. a
4. b

Critically Appraising the Literature Review
Correct answers include any of the following:
    a. Identify both primary and secondary sources.
    b. Are the studies current?
    c. What landmark studies are included?

d. Have the relevant studies been critically appraised?
e. Are relevant theories discussed?
f. Is the current knowledge summarized?
g. Are literature gaps or what is not known identified?
h. Is the review organized?
i. Is the review logical?
j. Are the studies paraphrased?

Performing Literature Searches

1. c
2. b
3. a, b, c, d
4. b
5. a
6. d
7. a, c
8. a
9. a, c
10. a, possibly c
11. AND
12. a. CINAHL
    b. OVID
    c. EBSCO
    d. MEDLINE

Writing a Review of Literature

a. Introduction previews the focus of the review, including the major areas to be covered in the literature review.
b. The section on Empirical Literature reviews and provides the critical appraisal of relevant studies. This provides the reader with the current knowledge of the field plus the gaps in prior studies.
c. The section on Theoretical Sources provides concepts and conceptual frameworks that provide knowledge to organize and support the study.
d. The Summary concludes the review by clearing indicating what is known and not known in the area of the study. This provides a basis to conduct the study.

Crossword Puzzle

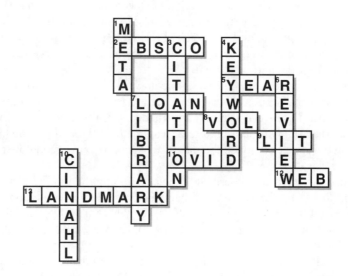

Exercises in Critical Appraisal

1. a. name of the journal
   b. year the study was published
   c. volume number of the journal
   d. pages of the article
   e. issue number of the journal
   f. Schachman
   g. Online fathering: The experience of first-time fatherhood in combat-deployed troops.
2. Padula, C. A., Yeaw, E., & Mistry, S. (2009). A home-based nurse-coached inspiratory muscle training intervention in heart failure. *Applied Nursing Research, 22,* 18-25.
3. a. title and pages of the article
   b. volume number of the journal and pages of the article
   c. year the article was published and volume and issue numbers of the journal
4. a. Literature Review
   b. Review of Literature
5. In the Introduction (not labeled) and in the Discussion
6. Yes, relevant studies are identified and described. By examining the literature review section and the references of the Padula et al. (2009) study, it appears that they identified and described at least eight relevant studies in their literature review:
   Cahalin, Semingran, & Dec (1997);
   Dall'Ago, Chiappa, Guths, Stein, & Ribeiro (2006);
   Johnson, Cowley, & Kinnear (1998);
   Laoutaris et al. (2004);
   Mancini, Henson, LaManca, Donchez, & Levine (1995);
   Martinez et al. (2001);
   Padula & Yeaw (2001);
   Weiner, Waizman, Magadle, Berar-Yanan, & Pelled (1999).
7. Padula et al. (2009) began the literature review by describing biological explanations for dyspnea. They cite Gibbs et al. (1990) as a source for hemodynamic and neurohormonal models. The muscle hypothesis was credited to Clark et al. (1996) and elaborated on by McConnell et al. (2003) and by Vibarel et al. (2002). They also base their study framework and intervention on Bandura's (1986) Self-Efficacy Theory.
8. theoretical source
9. primary
10. The Padula et al. study was published in 2009. The manuscript was first submitted in September 2006 and revised and accepted in February 2007. The references range from 1982 through 2006. It is apparent that the authors continued to search for new literature until the paper was submitted for publication. The sources cited were relevant to the topic or were necessary to provide justification for the methods used (i.e., instruments and scales). Of the 26 citations, only 10 (38%) were published in the 10 years prior to 2009 and only one (<4%) was published in the 5 years prior to 2009. However, 6 of the older citations were necessary to provide the theoretical perspective and 5 were cited related to measurement scales. Another issue to consider is that the authors could not add references after the manuscript was accepted for publication (2007). Thus, the references can be judged to be current.
11. A search of CINAHL would be needed. One was done in April 2010, limited to 2001-2010, used the phrase of HEART FAILURE as part of a subject heading. A second search was run with the same limiters using RESPIRATORY MUSCLES as part of a subject and yielded 483 hits. Combining the two searches yielded 21 hits. Of these 21 sources, only one appeared to be a study that might add to the knowledge on this topic, but the studies cited in the article comprise the majority of what is known about respiratory muscle training in heart failure patients.
12. Yes, relevant studies are identified and described. When examining the Bindler et al. (2007) Review of the Literature section and References, it can be seen that over 20 studies are cited. Some examples are: Falkner et al. (2002); Cook et al. (2003); de Ferranti et al. (2004); Golley et al. (2006); Steinberger & Daniels (2003); Duncan et al. (2004); Molnar (2004) Srinvasan et al. (1999); Fagot-Campagna et al. (2001); Valle et al. (2002).
13. The citations for the Bindler et al. (2007) article do not include any that are obviously theoretical or conceptual. In addition, this study has no identified framework. The theoretical knowledge basis for the study

seems to be physiological and pathological theory. This content is provided by the following sources: Kelley (2000), Ludwig et al. (1999), and Mayer-Davis et al. (1997).

14. secondary source, primary source

15. The Bindler et al. (2007) study has current sources. The references ranged from 1985 through 2006, and the article was published in early 2007. There is no indication when the article was submitted or accepted for publication. Of the 60 sources, 49 (82%), were published in the last 10 years, including 25 (42%) in the past 5 years.

16. Bindler et al. (2007) provided detailed coverage of relevant studies (pp. 202-206) and used tables to display diagnostic criteria that were used by the researchers. They concluded that the ethnic minority children are underrepresented in the studies that have been conducted. They noted that "more information is needed to establish the contribution of various characteristics to insulin resistance in children" (p. 206). The study was supported by a very strong review of the literature.

    A CINAHL search, limited to 2007-2010, was conducted using *metabolic syndrome*, *school children*, and *minority* as search terms. No additional studies were found.

17. Schachman (2010) cited studies about the father's presence during labor and the impact on maternal outcomes. The manuscript was accepted for publication in 2009. Some of the studies cited included Essex and Pickett (2008), Hodnet et al. (2007), Pleck and Masciadrelli (2004), and Premberg et al. (2008). Other citations referred to studies about fathers' feelings about being present: Deave and Johnson (2008), Johnson (2002), Rosich-Medina and Shetty (2007), Goodman (2005), and Jordan (1990). She concluded the short review of the literature that what was not known was the perspectives of fathers who are "absent during this important event" (p. 226).

18. Two theoretical or sociocultural analyses were included: Draper (2003) and Barclay and Lupton (1999).

19. secondary source, primary source

20. The references range from 1978 through 2009. The article was accepted in 2009 and published in 2010. Of the 17 studies cited, 13 (76%) were published in or after 2001, including 7 (41%) in or after 2006. Of the older citations, two were related to the research methods (Colaizzi, 1978; Streubert & Carpenter, 1999). The literature review is current.

21. A CINAHL search using *fathers* and *labor*, limited to 2008 through 2010, yielded four citations, three of which were studies published in 2009; the year the Schachman (2010) article was published. Because this is a phenomenological study, Schachman (2010) compares the findings to the research findings in the literature. The literature helps to link the new findings to the current literature, with Schachman (2010) providing a current picture of what is known about fathering for fathers absent because of deployment. Researchers building on her work would want to include the newer studies in their reviews of the literature.

CHAPTER 7—UNDERSTANDING THEORY AND RESEARCH FRAMEWORKS

Key Terms
1. g
2. e
3. a
4. d
5. b
6. j
7. k
8. c
9. h
10. f
11. i

Key Ideas
1. to organize what we know about a phenomenon and provide frameworks for studies
2. determining the accuracy of selected relational statements or propositions in a theory
3. conceptual models
4. framework
5. disconnected
6. the study framework
7. concepts
8. constructs
9. variable

10. propositions or relationships
11. hypotheses
12. diagram the concepts and their relationships to provide a framework for a study
13. the major concepts and the relationships among these concepts
14. research tradition
15. prescriptive
16. variable
17. concepts, definitions of concepts, propositions or relationships among the concepts, theory, and conceptual map
18. Critically appraising
19. implied
20. See Table 7-5 in *Understanding Nursing Research* for the names of a variety of middle-range theories used as frameworks in nursing studies
21. health promotion
22. Orem

Making Connections

Levels of Abstraction
Highest to lowest abstraction for the terms: construct, concept, variable, and operational definition

Elements of Theory
1. Physical health, psychological health, and quality of life
2. Relationships or propositions
3. Conceptual map for a study framework

Examples of Frameworks
1. f
2. h
3. g
4. c

5. e
6. a
7. d
8. b

Crossword Puzzle

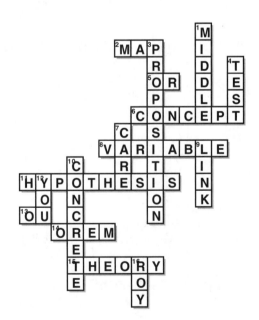

Exercises in Critical Appraisal

Critical Appraisal of Bindler, Massey, Shultz, Mills, and Short (2007) Study

1. Concepts:
    a. metabolic syndrome
    b. lifestyle factors
    c. environment
    d. genetic component
2. Conceptual definitions:
    a. metabolic syndrome—a syndrome typified by a decrease in the number of insulin receptors and in their functional ability at the cellular level (insulin resistance) with resultant hyperinsulinemia and development of type 2 diabetes
    b. lifestyle factors that lead to metabolic syndrome—high saturated fat and low-fiber diets, stress, and physical inactivity
    c. environment that leads to metabolic syndrome—limited opportunity for physical activity and access to fresh and nutritious food choices
    d. genetics—certain population groups, such as Native Americans and Hispanic Americans, are at higher risk for metabolic syndrome
3. Variables: glucose, total cholesterol (TC), high-density lipoprotein cholesterol (HDL-C), low-density lipoprotein cholesterol (LDL-C), triglycerides, insulin level, blood pressure, smoking history, physical fitness, body fat, diet, family history, population group/ethnicity.
4. Relationship between concepts and variables in the Bindler et al. (2007) study.

Concept	Variable
Metabolic syndrome	Glucose, TC, HDL-C, LDL-C, Triglycerides, Insulin level, Blood pressure
Lifestyle and environment	Smoking history, Physical fitness, Body fat, Diet
Genetics	Family history, Ethnicity

5. Link of concepts, variables, and measurement methods for Bindler et al. (2007) study.

Concept	Variable(s)	Measurement Method(s)
Metabolic syndrome	Glucose TC, HDL-C, LDL-C Triglycerides Insulin level Blood pressure	Blood draw Blood draw Blood draw Blood draw Cuff, stethoscope, and sphygmomanometer
Lifestyle and environment	Smoking history Physical fitness Body Fat Diet	Questionnaire Canadian Aerobic Fitness Test $\rightarrow$ VO$_{2max}$ Godon Leisure Time Questionnaire $\rightarrow$ MET Height & weight $\rightarrow$ BMI Calipers $\rightarrow$ Triceps skinfold thickness Youth/Adolescent Questionnaire (YAQ) Interview for 24 hr recall $\rightarrow$ Healthy Eating Index
Genetics	Family history Population group/ethnicity	Medical history form Parental interview/questionnaire

6. The study does not have a clearly identified framework but draws upon physiological and pathological theories as a theoretical basis for the study. However, the relevant concepts are clearly identified and defined in the study. Many of the variables are not conceptually defined but all the variables are operationally defined (see the table above that links concepts, variables, and measurement methods).

Critical Appraisal of Padula, Yeaw, and Mistry (2009) Study

1. Padula et al. (2009) had a clearly identified framework for their study. The researchers used Bandura's Self-Efficacy Theory to provide a framework for their study (see the Framework section in the article).

2. The major study concepts include: situational demands, vicarious experiences, verbal persuasion, enactive attainment, performance accomplishment, and enhanced self-efficacy.

3. "*Self-efficacy* refers to people's belief in their capabilities to mobilize the motivation, cognitive resources, and course of action needed to meet given situational demands" (p. 218).

4. The independent variable is nurse-coached inspiratory muscle training (IMT). The dependent variables are: inspiratory muscle strength (IMS); dyspnea; dyspnea intensity and distress; self-efficacy related to breathing (CSES); physical/functional and psychosocial health-related quality of life (HRQOL); and clinical assessment variables (weight, blood pressure, pulse, respiratory rate, respiratory pattern, edema, and lung sounds).

5. Link of concepts to variables are presented in the table below.

Concept	Variable(s)
Situational demands	Dyspnea Dyspnea intensity and distress
Vicarious experiences Verbal persuasion Enactive attainment	Nurse-coached inspiratory muscle training (IMT) intervention
Performance accomplishment Enhanced self-efficacy	IMS Self-efficacy related to breathing Physical/functional and psychosocial HRQOL Clinical assessment variables (weight, blood pressure, pulse, respiratory rate, respiratory pattern, edema, and lung sounds)

6. Link of concepts, variables, and measurement methods are presented in the table below.

Concept	Variable(s)	Measurement Method(s) for Dependent Variables and Manipulation of Independent Variable
Situational demands	Dyspnea Dyspnea intensity and distress	Measured with Borg scale Chronic Respiratory Disease Questionnaire (CRDQ)
Vicarious experiences Verbal persuasion Enactive attainment	Nurse-coached inspiratory muscle training (IMT) intervention	IMT is the study treatment or intervention that was manipulated or implemented in the study and is described in detail in the article.
Performance accomplishment Enhanced self-efficacy	Self-efficacy related to breathing Physical/functional and psychosocial health-related quality of life Clinical assessment variables (weight, blood pressure, pulse, respiratory rate, respiratory pattern, edema, and lung sounds)	COPD Self-Efficacy Scale (CSES) Medical Outcomes Study (MOS) Health-Related Quality of Life (HRQOL) Scale Home visit by nurse with standard clinical measurement of the clinical assessment variables

7. No, Padula et al. (2009) did not provide a map or model of their study framework.

CHAPTER 8—CLARIFYING QUANTITATIVE RESEARCH DESIGNS

Key Terms

1. a
2. g
3. b
4. l
5. d
6. c
7. k

8. j
9. f
10. n
11. i
12. e
13. h
14. m

Key Ideas

1. effects or outcomes
2. cause, effect, cause
3. biases or extraneous variables
4. control
5. treatment, intervention, or independent variable
6. design validity
7. cause and effect, causality, or the effect of a treatment on a study outcome
8. multicausality
9. bias or error or threats to design validity
10. control
11. experimental design
12. descriptive or correlational studies
13. comparative descriptive
14. correlational
15. middle-range theories
16. error or bias
17. You might include any of the following:
    a. random assignment of subjects to groups
    b. manipulation of independent variable by researcher
    c. control of the setting
    d. include a control or comparison group
    e. control of extraneous variables
    f. random selection of subjects if possible
18. control
19. large
20. You might include any of the following:
    a. physiological
    b. psychological
    c. social
    d. educational
    e. environmental
    f. combination of the above

Making Connections

Control and Designs for Nursing Studies

1. Randomized clinical trial—testing the effectiveness of a new hypertensive medication.
   Study has a large sample size with random assignment to the comparison and experimental groups. In addition, the medication is manipulated and controlled including dose, route, and time.
2. Quasi-experimental design—used to examine the effect of a new pain scoring system. The children in the experimental group received the new scoring system, and the children in the comparison group had the old scoring system.
   The treatment of the scoring system is controlled as is the age of the children. The children were obtained by a sample of convenience and were not randomly assigned to groups but the groups were equal in number.

3. Case study—to gain an in-depth understanding of the nursing class.
    There is no control, only a description of the sample as it exists in a natural setting.
4. Descriptive survey design—nurses were surveyed to determine their attitudes toward home hemodialysis.
    No controls were identified for this descriptive study, which is common.
5. Replication study—repeating a previous study to determine the consistency in the results from one study to another.
    Controls in the replication masters' thesis study would be consistent with the initial study.
6. Descriptive study—identifying and describing the health promotion behaviors of patients experiencing their first myocardial infarction (MI).
    The only control is the limitation of sample to patients with first MI.
7. Comparative descriptive design—examining the differences between males' and females' health promotion behaviors.
    The study population is people with diabetes. No controls are implemented in this study.
8. Quasi-experimental design with two posttests—examining the effects of vitamins on weight gain at 6 months and 1 year for infants with failure to thrive.
    The treatment of vitamins is controlled and manipulated in this study to determine the effect on weight gain. Two posttests were conducted because weight gain was measured at 6 months and 1 year. The sample was one of convenience, and the groups were based on the primary practice sites. The subjects were not randomly assigned to groups.
9. Model testing design—testing the use of the Orem Self-Care Model to predict self-care behaviors in diabetic adolescents.
    There is no indication of control being implemented in this study.
10. Experimental study design—study examines the effect of a new chemotherapy agent on tumor size.
    Study control is indicated by random sample, random assignment to groups, controlled treatment, controlled measurement of tumor size, and control of data collection process.

Mapping the Design

1. The focus of a descriptive study design is to describe selected variables in the sample. The map of the descriptive design is found in Figure 8-3, page 259 of your textbook.
2. The focus of a descriptive correlational design is to examine relationships among variables in a single sample. The map for this design is found in Figure 8-6, page 256 of your textbook.
3. The quasi-experimental design usually has a sample of convenience with random assignment to groups. Sometimes the groups are determined based on the setting and are not randomly assigned to the experimental and comparison groups. The map for this study design is found in Figure 8-11, page 275 of your textbook.

Crossword Puzzle

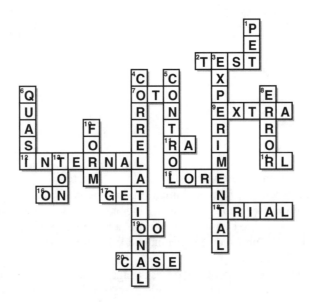

Exercises in Critical Appraisal

Answers address the critical appraisal of the design of the Bindler et al. (2007) study in Appendix B.

1. Bindler et al.'s (2007) study has a predictive correlational design.
2. Group comparisons: Bindler et al.'s (2007) study mainly focused on relationships but did make comparisons among three ethnic groups, Native American, Hispanic, and Caucasian groups, on:
   a. Demographic variables (i.e. age, sex, family history) (see Table 3, p. 207)
   b. Physical fitness variables (i.e., VO_{2max}, MET score) (see Table 3)
   c. Smoking history (see Table 3)
   d. BP (see Table 3)
   e. Measures of body fat (i.e., ht., wt., BMI, skinfold percentile) (see Table 3)
   f. Biophysiological measures of serum cholesterol, triglycerides, and glucose (see Table 4, p. 208)
   g. Multiple dietary intake factors (e.g., carbohydrates, proteins, total fat, saturated fat… fiber (see Table 4)
   h. Some other comparisons were made on the insulin levels of different genders and age groups.
3. You might have identified any of the following strengths of the design for the Bindler et al. (2007) study.
   a. Data collected at one time in same setting.
   b. Subjects obtained from a racially mixed population.
   c. Sample size of Hispanics is strong but the numbers of Native Americans and Caucasians were limited.
   d. Content experts (e.g., dietitian) used to collect data related to their expertise.
   e. Training of data collectors.
   f. Objective measurement of many variables with physiological measurement methods, such as insulin levels, cholesterol values, blood pressure.
   g. Multiple methods used to measure some variables.
   h. Steps were taken with data collection to ensure accuracy and precision of physiological measures and reliability and validity of the diet data.
4. Sources of bias: You might have identified any of the following ideas or you might have identified other biases in the Bindler et al. (2007) study.
   a. Used only subject recall for measuring diet intake, possibly leading to mono-method bias or only one method being used to measure the variable (in addition, subject recall has been criticized as not accurately reflecting diet intake).
   b. The sample was not randomly selected; it was a nonprobability sample of convenience. The parents volunteered for the study in response to a flyer sent home with their children and they may be different from those who did not volunteer (e.g., must have been able to read the flyer). However, the researchers provided the flyer in both English and Spanish to increase the representativeness of the sample.
   c. Only children with no identified illnesses or medications were included—the sample, therefore, did not represent the population, which would include children with identified illnesses.
   d. No power analysis was addressed to determine the sample size needed for the study. Was the sample size large enough to prevent a Type II error? What was the effect size for the study?
   e. Only 88 of the 100 subjects identified their ethnicity and the sample included 64 Hispanics, 15 Native Americans, and 9 Caucasians. The group sizes for the Native Americans and Caucasians are really too low for this study.
5. Methods of control: Identify any three of the following methods of control in the Bindler et al. (2007) study.
   a. Controlling measurement: Blood pressures were measured the same way three times and the average value was used.
   b. Controlling extraneous variables: Blood draws were done in early morning by licensed phlebotomist after the subjects had fasted for 10 hours.
   c. Controlling environment: All measurements were completed in 1 day at the same setting.
   d. Controlling measurement reliability: Interrater reliability was established among all researchers by training and evaluating them for reliability on measurement and for assistance to children during questionnaire completion.
   e. Controlling mono-operation bias: Used multiple measures for each variable.
   f. Controlling for the effects of maturation: Fed students after fasting blood draws so that increasing hunger did not affect study results.

g.   Controlling analysis: Completed questionnaires were returned to YAQ developers at the Harvard School of Public Health for the calculation of the dietary intake of nutrients and percentage of recommended dietary allowance (RDA) for each nutrient.

6.   Populations generalized to in the Bindler et al. (2007) study. Generalization is limited to ethnically mixed populations of children in 4th–8th grades who live in small rural farm communities with limited access to fast-food and who speak and write English or Spanish. The small number of Caucasians (9 subjects) and Native Americans (15 subjects) included in the study limit the generalizability of the findings to these two ethnic groups. Study findings really are best generalized to Hispanics.

Answers address the critical appraisal of the design of the Padula, Yeaw, and Mistry (2009) study found in Appendix B.

1.   Type of Design: "Two-group quasi-experimental design with random assignment to groups" (Padula et al., 2009, p. 20).

2.   Comparisons were made in the Padula et al. (2009) study and are described as follows.

Because this was a quasi-experimental study focused on determining the effects of a treatment on selected dependent variables, the experimental and the control groups were compared on: inspiratory muscle strength (IMS), dyspnea, physical/functional and psychosocial health-related quality of life (HRQOL), self-efficacy, BP, HR, and respiratory rate. In addition, "baseline scores, including the MOS SF-36 (HRQOL), self-efficacy, CRDQ (dyspnea), diastolic and systolic BP, and HR, were comparable in the two groups; there were no statistically significant differences" (Padula et al., 2009, p. 291). These comparisons were done on the pretests for both the treatment and the control groups indicating that the groups were alike at the start of the study, which is a strength of this design.

3.   Strengths in the Padula et al. (2009) study design include any of the following:
a.   Random assignment to experimental and control groups using a toss of a coin.
b.   Structured inspiratory muscle training (IMT) intervention that was based on Bandura's theory of self-efficacy.
c.   Research assistants (RAs) were trained for consistent implementation of the treatment and measurement of the dependent variables.
d.   Quality sampling inclusion and exclusion criteria to decrease potential extraneous variables.
e.   Strictly following the sampling criteria for inclusion in the study.
f.   Quality measurement methods for measuring IMS, dyspnea, and other physiological variables (BP, HR, and RR).
g.   Detailed plan for implementing the study to decrease the potential for bias.
h.   Pretests of experimental and control groups' dependent variables to ensure the groups were similar at the start of the study.

4.   Potential sources of bias you might have identified in the Padula et al. (2009) study include the following:
a.   The original sample was not random and there is a potential for sampling bias with a nonprobability sample of convenience.
b.   The final sample size was small with 32 subjects and there were some nonsignificant findings so there was a potential for a Type II error because of small sample size.
c.   The instruments used to measure physical/functional and psychosocial HRQOL and self-efficacy might have lacked validity for this population of heart failure patients.
d.   The patient logs and diaries were useful, but were not universally used in the study.
e.   Subjective reporting of activities that caused shortness of breath.

5.   Methods of control used in the Padula et al. (2009) study design that you might have identified include the following:
a.   Extensive control of the IMT intervention and RAs ensured the subjects complied with the treatment.
b.   Control of the implementation of the sampling criteria.
c.   Control of the measurement of the physiological variables of dyspnea, IMS, HR, BP, and RR.
d.   Control of the ethical aspects of the study such as institutional board review approval and obtaining informed consent from the subjects.

6.   The researchers generalized the effectiveness of the IMT for use in patients with HF. The IMT intervention improved the patients' physical functioning but not their HRQOL or self-efficacy. Additional research is needed to determine the effectiveness of the IMT on these variables.

CHAPTER 9—EXAMINING POPULATIONS AND SAMPLES IN RESEARCH

Key Terms

1. j
2. a
3. n
4. g
5. k
6. f
7. m
8. i
9. l
10. b
11. d
12. e
13. h
14. c
15. o

Key Ideas

1. elements
2. target population
3. sample, accessible population, and target population
4. You might identify any two of the following:
   a. Compare the demographic characteristics of the sample with those of the target population determined from previous research.
   b. Compare mean sample values of study variables with the values of the target population determined from previous research.
   c. Determine sample attrition rate and identify the reasons for the attrition or withdrawal of subjects from the study.
   d. Evaluate the possibilities of systematic bias in the sample in terms of the setting, characteristics of the sample, and ranges of values on measured variables.
   e. Identify the refusal rate in the study and identify the reasons potential subjects refused to participate.
5. the expected difference in values that occurs when different subjects from the same sample are examined
6. sampling frame
7. strategies used to obtain a sample for a study
8. You might choose any of the following:
   a. Was the sampling plan adequately identified?
   b. Did the researcher successfully implement the sampling plan?
   c. Was the sampling plan effective in achieving representativeness of the target population?
   d. Were the subjects selected from a sampling frame?
   e. Were the subjects randomly selected?
9. homogeneous
10. heterogeneous
11. sampling criteria
12. sample characteristics
13. sample attrition or mortality
14. random
15. nonrandom or nonprobability
16. a. simple random sampling
    b. stratified random sampling
    c. cluster sampling
    d. systematic sampling
17. probability or random
18. a. convenience sampling
    b. quota sampling
    c. purposive sampling
    d. network sampling
19. nonprobability
20. accidental sampling
21. judgmental sampling
22. power analysis

23. differences or relationships
24. 0.8 or 80%
25. power analysis
26. null hypothesis
27. a. effect size of a study
    b. type of study
    c. number of variables
    d. measurement sensitivity
    e. data analysis techniques
28. a. natural setting
    b. partially controlled setting
    c. highly controlled setting
29. inclusion and exclusion
30. Refusal rate = 33 refused ÷ 250 subjects approached = 0.132 x 100% = 13.2%

Making Connections

Sampling Methods for Quantitative and Qualitative Studies

1. f
2. b
3. c
4. a
5. b
6. g
7. h
8. b
9. e
10. d

11. f
12. c
13. d
14. b
15. f
16. h
17. i
18. a
19. d
20. b

Determining Sample Size for Quantitative and Qualitative Research

1. a
2. c
3. b
4. a
5. b

6. b
7. c
8. b
9. a
10. b

Crossword Puzzle

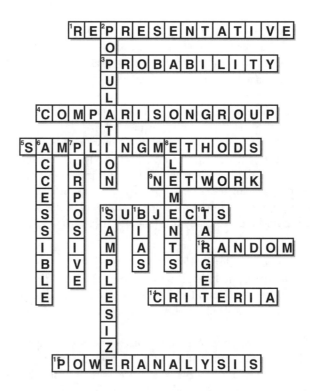

Exercises in Critical Appraisal

Bindler et al. (2007) Study

1. Population was school-age children.
2. Inclusion sample criteria were: Children "attending fourth to eighth grades at public elementary and middle schools" and "Participants who spoke English or Spanish were eligible" (p. 205). Exclusion sample criteria: Children with identified illnesses or on medications were excluded.
3. In the Results section of the study was a subsection entitled "Description of Sample" that identified the sample characteristics for the study, as well as Table 3 (p. 207) in the study. "The age range of the sample was 9-15 years (M = 12 years). The sample included 52 boys and 48 girls. Sixty-four (64%) claimed to be purely Hispanic, 15 (15%) claimed to be purely Native American, and 9 (9%) claimed to be purely Caucasian. Twelve (12%) additional subjects claimed to have mixed-race ethnic heritage. All Hispanic children had Mexico as origin of the family and were employed in farming or food processing industries. There were no significant differences among ethnic groups regarding age or gender; reported family history of cardiovascular disease, diabetes, overweight, or smoking; physical activity; weight percentiles; BMI percentiles; or triceps skin fold percentiles. Table 3 shows the demographic data and physical measurements of the total sample and of the ethnic subsample (those children identifying with just one major ethnic group)" (Bindler et al., 2007, p. 206) (see Table 3 in the article in Appendix B on p. 207).
4. Sample size was "100 children (representing approximately 15% of eligible students) attending fourth to eighth grades at public elementary and middle schools" (p. 205). No power analysis was mentioned to determine sample size.
5. The adequacy of the sample size is questionable because the researchers conducted analyses on small groups formed based on ethnic origin with only 15 Native Americans, 9 Caucasians, and 12 mixed race. Some of the study results were not significant, which might be because of an inadequate sample size and would be considered a Type II error. Sample size is also limited for the large number of variables that are examined in this study. The lack of a power analysis to determine the sample size limits the ability of the reader to judge the adequacy of a sample.
6. The sample attrition or mortality was not discussed in this study but the researchers did mention in the Results section that blood samples were not obtained on two children so they were omitted from this aspect of the analyses. This study would have been strengthened by a discussion of sample attrition and a rationale for why the subjects dropped out of the study.

7. Nonprobability sampling.
8. The sampling method is a convenience or accidental sampling method.
9. The representativeness of the sample is limited because only 15% of the eligible students attending the public elementary and middle schools participated. The researchers did not address acceptance rate or the attrition rate, which would have been useful in determining the representativeness of the sample. The sample included 64 Hispanic students, which is more representative for that group than for the Caucasians with 9 subjects and the Native Americans with 15 subjects. Based on the information provided, the representativeness of the sample of the target population is limited.
10. The generalization of the study findings is decreased by the nonprobability sampling method and the limited representativeness of the sample for selected ethnic groups. However, because some of these study findings were consistent with the findings of other studies, this increases the generalizability of the findings. Because this is a relatively new area of research for children, the findings can be generalized to the sample and probably the accessible population but not to the target population. Additional research is needed in this problem area before the findings are ready for generalization.

Padula et al. (2009) Study
1. The population is adults with heart failure (HF).
2. Sampling criteria: "Inclusion criteria included the following: (1) adult; (2); community dwelling; (3) stable Class II or III HF with an ejection fraction of <45%; (4) without coexisting pulmonary disease; and (5) without cognitive impairment as measured by Mini Mental Status Exam" (p. 220). Subjects were excluded because of the COPD comorbidity.
3. Sample characteristics: "The demographic characteristics of the two groups are illustrated in Table 1 (p. 221). The mean age was 74.7 years, ranging from 32 to 95 years for both groups. The gender (47% male) and ethnicity (85% white, 9% Hispanic, 3% Black, and 3% Native American) of the sample corresponded closely to those of the state population (48% male, 87% White, and 13% non-White), with the minority population slightly overrepresented in the study. The NYHA [New York Heart Association] classification among the total sample was 51.8% Class II and 48.3% Class III" (p. 221). Additional demographic or sample characteristics for the study groups (treatment and control) are shown in Table 1." See article in Appendix B for Table 1 on p. 221.
4. A total of 288 subjects were screened and 248 (86%) were ineligible or did not meet the sample criteria to participate in the study. Forty (13.9%) of the subjects screened were eligible for the study and four (10%) refused to participate in the study. The researchers included a recruitment flowchart in their study to clarify the sampling process but the number of subjects eligible for the study was 40 instead of the 36 identified in the figure (see Figure 1, p. 220).
5. Sample size: The original sample size was approximately 36 subjects but only 32 subjects completed the study with 15 subjects in the treatment group and 17 in the control group. The researchers need to clarify the size of the original sample.
6. No power analysis was done to determine the sample size needed for the study. The sample size was adequate to determine significant differences between the treatment and control groups for the inspiratory muscle strength, dyspnea, and respiratory rate. However, no significant differences were found between the groups for the self-efficacy and physical/functional and psychosocial dimensions of health-related quality of life. This lack of significance could have been because of inadequate sample size (Type II error) or measurement problems as indicated by the researchers.
7. One subject moved from the treatment to the control group and two (6%) of the subjects withdrew from the study.
8. nonprobability sample
9. convenience sampling
10. The sample was not random, which decreases its probability of being representative of the target population. However, the researchers indicated that the distribution of gender and ethnicity in the sample closely corresponded to those of the state population, which increased the representativeness of the sample.
11. Because the sample is nonrandom and the sample size is small, the researchers probably need to limit the generalization of their findings to the accessible population.

Schachman (2010) Study

1. The population was first-time fathers who were combat-deployed troops during the birth of their child.
2. Sample criteria: "Eligible participants were men stationed in Okinawa, Japan, who were attending a postdeployment briefing and self-identified as first-time fathers" (Schachman, 2010, p. 12).
3. Sample characteristics: "Duration of the combat deployment ranged from 6 to 10 months, and all men reported the birth of a first child during the deployment. Interviews were conducted within 1 month of their return, at which time the newborns were 2 to 6 months of age. All of the men were married and had a minimum of a high school education. Nearly 60% ($n = 10$) had at least 2 years of college. The mean age was 23 years ($SD = 2.3$; range = 19 to 26 years). Racial and ethnic breakdown was as follows: 10 Caucasians (59%), 4 African Americans (23%), 2 Hispanic (12%), and 1 other (6%)" (p. 227).
4. Sample size was 17 participants. No power analysis was conducted because this is a qualitative study, and sample size is determined by factors other than a power analysis (Burns & Grove, 2009).
5. The sample size seems adequate for this phenomenological study because recruitment of participants continued until saturation of data was achieved.
6. No sample attrition was mentioned.
7. Nonprobability sampling method was used in the study.
8. "Purpose sampling was used for recruitment of eligible participants" (p. 226).
9. Representativeness of the sample is not a focus of qualitative research. The focus is on understanding the specific study subjects.
10. Generalization of findings is not the focus of qualitative research. The focus is on understanding the phenomenon of first-time fatherhood of combat-deployed troops in this selected group of study participants.

CHAPTER 10—CLARIFYING MEASUREMENT AND DATA COLLECTION IN QUANTITATIVE RESEARCH

Key Terms

Measurement Concepts and Methods

1. g
2. m
3. i
4. e
5. k
6. h
7. o
8. a
9. d
10. c
11. b
12. n
13. f
14. j
15. l

Data Collection

1. d
2. b
3. c
4. e
5. f
6. a

Key Ideas

1. ratio level of measurement
2. 0.8
3. exhaustive and exclusive
4. unequal, equal
5. Likert
6. ratio
7. 1.00
8. developed
9. Cronbach's alpha
10. it is not valid

11. reliability and validity
12. unstructured
13. structured
14. Personal interview
15. Consistency
16. rating
17. visual analog scale
18. You might have listed any of the following or might have another idea that results in measurement error.
    a. Variations in administration of the measurement method.
    b. Subjects completing a paper-and-pencil scale accidentally marking the wrong column.
    c. Subjects misreading an item on a measurement method.
    d. Subjects leaving an item blank accidentally on a measurement scale.
    e. Punching the wrong key when entering data into the computer.
    f. Physiological measurement method that lacks precision and accuracy, like inaccurate blood pressure equipment.
    g. Poorly constructed scale or questionnaire that lacks reliability and validity.
19. a. Selecting subjects
    b. Collecting data in a consistent way
    c. Maintaining research controls indicated by the study design
    d. Protecting the study integrity (or validity)
    e. Solving problems that threaten to disrupt the study
20. serendipity

Making Connections

Measurement Error
1. b
2. b
3. a
4. b
5. a

Levels of Measurement
1. c
2. a
3. b
4. d
5. a
6. b
7. d
8. a
9. b or c
10. d
11. d
12. d
13. b
14. b or c
15. d
16. d
17. d
18. a
19. b
20. a

Scales
1. a. Likert scale
2. c. Visual analog scale
3. b. Rating scale

Sensitivity and Specificity
1.

Diagnostic Test Results	Disease Present	Disease not Present or Absent
Positive Test	*a* (true positive)	*b* (false positive)
Negative Test	*c* (false negative)	*d* (true negative)

2. Formula for sensitivity: $a/(a + c)$ = True positive rate
3. Formula for specificity: $d/(b + d)$ = True negative rate
4. 10%
5. 15%
6. Sensitivity = 90%/(90% + 15%) = 85.7%
7. Specificity = 85%/(10% + 85%) = 89.5%

Crossword Puzzle

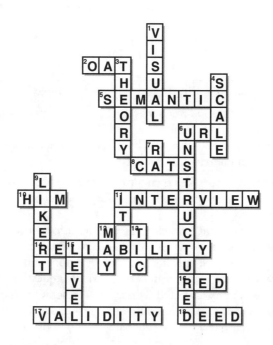

Exercises in Critical Appraisal

Bindler, Massey, Shultz, Mills, and Short (2007) study measurement methods and data collection are critically appraised with the following questions.
1. Bindler et al. (2007) study: Measurement methods and directness of measurement.

Variable(s)	Measurement Method(s)	Direct or Indirect Measurement Method
Glucose	Blood draw	Direct measurement
TC, HDL-C, LDL-C	Blood draw	Direct measurement
Blood pressure	Cuff, stethoscope, and sphygmomanometer	Direct measurement
Smoking history	Questionnaire	Indirect measurement
Body Fat	Height & weight → BMI	Indirect measurement
Diet	Youth/Adolescent Questionnaire (YAQ) Interview for 24 hr recall → Healthy Eating Index	Indirect measurement

2. Bindler et al. (2007) study: Precision and accuracy of measurement methods.

Variable(s) and Measurement Methods	Precision and Accuracy Information from Study
Glucose: Blood Draw	"Blood draws were completed in the early morning by the licensed phlebotomist after the children had fasted for at least 10 hours" (precision and accuracy) (Bindler, 2007, p. 205)
Blood pressure (BP): Cuff, stethoscope, and sphygmomanometer	"BP was measured on the right arm at heart level while the children were sitting; three readings were made with a 5-minute rest in between, and the mean of the three readings was used in analysis" (precision and accuracy) (Bindler, 2007, p. 205)

3. Bindler et al. (2007) description of the blood draws for glucose supported the precision and accuracy of the measurement of this variable. However, the authors might have provided more detail about the laboratory analysis of the blood and the reporting of the glucose values. The description of BP readings was excellent and indicates these readings were precise and accurate.
4. Bindler et al. (2007) identification of validity and reliability of the YAQ and smoking history questionnaire.

Questionnaire	Reliability and Validity Information from the Study
Diet: YAQ Questionnaire	YAQ is 151-item food frequency questionnaire, used with children from 8-18 years (reliability & validity), correlates well (0.54) (convergent validity) with 24-hour diet recalls, and used Statistical Analysis System to calculate means and standard deviations for energy and nutrients (reliability & validity).
Smoking History Questionnaire	Questionnaire that asked if children were current smokers or if they had ever tried smoking. No reliability or validity information about questionnaire.

5. Bindler et al. (2007) provided some solid reliability and validity information for the YAQ questionnaire supporting its use with children, its convergent validity, and quality statistical calculation of energy and nutrients. The smoking history questionnaire only includes two questions and the authors provide no information on the reliability and validity of this questionnaire. These two questions are a weak measure of smoking history that has questionable reliability and validity based on the subjects' recall.
6. Bindler et al. (2007) study was conducted to describe serum insulin levels and to investigate their relationships to metabolic syndrome criteria in a multiethnic sample of school children. These researchers provided a detailed description of data collection in the section entitled "Procedures and Instruments" in their study. "Study personnel consisted of a registered nurse/nutrition doctoral student, eight baccalaureate nursing students, a phlebotomist, one dietitian, and one dietetics student. All were trained and evaluated for reliability on measurement and for assistance to children during questionnaire completion. All measurements and questionnaires involving the children were implemented within a single day in the children's schools...

Parents of children in the study completed a medical family history form (accomplished during the informational evening session, or accomplished and sent later)... All forms were available in English and Spanish languages.

Blood draws were completed in the early morning by the licensed phlebotomist after the children had fasted for at least 10 hours; children were then fed breakfast before completing the remainder of the testing... Insulin was measured by solid-phase radioimmunoassay with the Coat-A-Count Insulin System (Diagnostic Products, Los Angeles, CA)...

Dietary data were collected by the use of the Youth/Adolescent Question (YAQ) (Rockett et al., 1997; Rockett & Colditz, 1997). This 151-item food frequency questionnaire has been used with children from 8 to 18 years and correlated well (0.54) with 24-hour diet recall results. It uses the Statistical Analysis System and calculates means and standard deviations for energy and all nutrients... In addition, a 24-hour diet recall was completed verbally with each child by a trained dietitian. These results were used to calculate Healthy Eating Index (HEI) scores... The 10 HEI scores are for grains, vegetables, fruit, milk, meat, total fat, saturated fat, cholesterol, sodium, and variety (Bowman, Lino, Gerrior, & Basiotis, 1998; Kennedy, Ohls, Carlson, & Fleming, 1995; Variyam, Smallwood, & Basiotis, 1998)." (Bindler et al., 2007, p. 205)

7. Bindler et al. (2007) provide excellent detail about the measurement methods (questionnaires and physiological measures) and how data were collected with these methods. The consistency of data collection was promoted with the use of highly qualified professionals who were trained for reliability in the data collection process. The forms and questionnaires were in both English and Spanish to increase the understanding of the subjects (both parents and children) and decrease possible errors in the data collected. The accuracy and precision of the physiologic methods were discussed in detail. One area of concern is the validity of the smoking history and dietary information because they were based on recall. The researchers tried to improve the quality of the dietary information by using the YAQ and conducting the 24-hour diet recall through interview with a trained dietitian. Another concern is the small number of subjects in the Caucasian (9 subjects) group and the Native American (15 subjects) group, which decreases the ability to generalize the study findings. However, this study does demonstrate quality in the measurement methods implemented and the process for collecting data.

Padula, Yeaw, and Mistry (2009) study measurement methods and data collection are critically appraised with the following questions.

1. Padula et al. (2009) measurement methods and directness of measurement.

Variable(s)	Measurement Method(s)	Direct or Indirect Measurement Method
Inspiratory muscle strength (IMS)	"IMS was measured by obtaining PI_{max} scores according to the universally accepted Black and Hyatt (1969) techniques." (p. 220)	Direct measurement
Self-efficacy	COPD Self-efficacy Scale (CSES)	Indirect measurement

2. Padula et al. (2009) precision and accuracy information for IMS.

Variable(s) and Measurement Methods	Precision (Reliability) and Accuracy (Validity) Information from Study
Inspiratory muscle strength (IMS): measured by PI_{max} scores	"IMS was measured by obtaining PI_{max} scores according to the universally accepted Black and Hyatt (1969) techniques [precision & accuracy]. PI_{max} is the maximal vacuum pressure generated at the mouth against an occluded airway that is sustained for one full second. The validity of the PI_{max} as a measure of IMS is supported by strong correlations between PI_{max} and maximal transdiaphragmatic pressure at $r + .93$ [convergent validity] (Braun, Arora, & Rochester, 1982). The PI_{max} has high test-retest reliability ($r - .97$ [$df + 89$]) if sufficient practice is provided to overcome learning effects (Larson et al., 2002). The test-retest reliability of the two inspiratory force meters (using $n = 12$) was established by the investigators at $r = .98$, using a minimum of five trials to obtain the average score for PI_{max}" [precision or reliability] (p. 220).

3. Padula et al. (2009) provided excellent detail about the precision (reliability) and accuracy (validity) of the measurement of IMS. The measurement techniques were implemented using a universally accepted process. The PI_{max} has very strong convergent validity ($r = .93$) when compared with another measurement technique. The test-retest reliability was also strong and detailed in the article.

4. Padula et al. (2009) study validity and reliability for CSES.

Scale	Reliability and Validity Information from the Study
CSES	CSES is a "34-item measure with good test-retest reliability ($r + 0.77$) and excellent internal consistency (Cronbach's $\alpha = .95$) [reliability] (Wigal, Creer, & Kostes, 1991). Because this scale was used primarily with patients with COPD, we submitted it to a panel of experts to confirm its content validity for use in an HF [heart failure] sample. Ten advanced-practice nurses experienced in HF management responded to the questionnaire. Findings were supportive of using the CSES, with modification of the content 'when I am' to 'when I *feel*' in six items [construct validity]. The scale was then piloted using a representative sample of people with HF" [validity and reliability] (p. 221).

5. The CSES has very strong reliability for use with COPD patients and this was documented in the article but the authors did not discuss the reliability of the scale for HF patients. A Cronbach's alpha should have been run on the scale for the sample in this study. In addition, the scale was pilot tested using a representative sample but there is no mention of the reliability of the scale from the pilot. The authors only discuss the content validity of the scale for use with HF patients and this validity seems adequate. But additional validity information is needed about this scale and whether it measures self-efficacy in HF patients. The study results were not significant in this area and that might be because of the limitations (reliability and validity) of the CSES in measuring self-efficacy in HF patients.

6. Padula et al. (2009) data collection process is presented in detail under the headings of "Recruitment" and "Measures." The recruitment sites included physicians' offices, home-care agencies, provider referral, and newspaper advertisement. The measurement of IMS was detailed in question 4 above. "*Dyspnea* was measured by the Borg (1982) scale, which incorporates the use of category methods with ratio properties... *Dyspnea intensity and distress* were operationalized using the dyspnea scale of the CRDQ (Guyatt, Berman, Townsend, Pugsley, & Chambers, 1987). The CRDQ elicits subjects' shortness of breath (SOB) due to activities... *Physical/functional and psychosocial dimensions of HRQOL* were measured by the MOS SF-36 (Ware & Sherbourne, 1992)... General *demographic data* and *New York Heart Association (NYHA) classification*, a widely used system to classify limitations in ability to perform physical activity were obtained at baseline. *Clinical assessments* during home visits included weight, HR, BP, RR, and respiratory pattern, edema, lung sounds, and review of self-reported symptoms. A log was used to collect and document data at baseline, Week 1, Week 3, Week 6, Week 9, and Week 12" (p. 221).

7 Padula et al. (2009) provided extensive discussion of the data collection process. The recruitment of subjects is discussed in detail followed by a strong discussion of how study variables were measured with a variety of measurement methods. The authors also discussed the ethical precautions that they took related to the study. "This study was reviewed and approved by three institutional review boards. Recruiting physicians signed the Federal Wide Assurance forms, and RAs (research assistants) completed human subjects' certifications" (p. 220). The authors also detailed the implementation of the study treatment of the inspiratory muscle training (IMT) program.

CHAPTER 11—UNDERSTANDING STATISTICS IN RESEARCH

Key Terms

1. o
2. l
3. g
4. n
5. e
6. m
7. c
8. j

9. a
10. h
11. f
12. d
13. i
14. b
15. k

Key Ideas

1. a. significant and predicted results
   b. nonsignificant results
   c. significant and unpredicted results
   d. mixed results
   e. unexpected results
2. a. findings
   b. conclusions
   c. significance of findings
   d. generalization of findings
   e. implications of the findings for practice
   f. suggestions for further study
3. You might have listed any of the following:
   a. preparing the data for analysis

    b. describing the sample
    c. testing the reliability of the measurement methods
    d. conducting exploratory analysis of the data
    e. conducting confirmatory analyses guided by objectives, questions, or hypotheses
    f. conducting post hoc analyses
4. reduce and organize numerical data from a study to give it meaning.
5. You could have listed any three of the following:
    a. Estimates of central tendency are calculated for variables relevant to describing the sample, such as mode, median, and mean.
    b. Estimates of dispersion are calculated for variables relevant to describing the sample, such as range, variance, and standard deviation.
    c. Data are examined on each variable using measures of central tendency and dispersion to determine variation in the data and to identify outliers.
    d. Frequencies and percentages are calculated for nominal and ordinal data to determine the occurrence of demographic variables. For example, with a sample size of 220, the sample was 121 (55%) female and 99 (45%) male.
    e. Relationships among variables relevant to the sample are examined.
    f. Differences among groups are examined to demonstrate equivalence of study groups.
6. The normal curve is a symmetrical curve where the mean, median, and mode fall at the same point. See Figure 12-1, p. 435 in your textbook for a drawing of the normal curve.
7. 95%
8. one-tailed test of significance
9. Type I error
10. ANOVA
11. mode
12. the group size
13. skewed
14. scatterplot
15. bivariate

Making Connections

Linking Statistics with Analysis Techniques

1.	b	6.	a
2.	e	7.	d
3.	j	8.	g
4.	c	9.	h
5.	f	10.	i

Linking Level of Measurement with Analysis Techniques

1.	c	9.	c
2.	a	10.	b & c
3.	c	11.	a
4.	c	12.	a & b
5.	a & b	13.	c
6.	b	14.	c
7.	c	15.	a & b
8.	c		

Statements, Inferences, and Generalizations

1. d
2. b
3. a
4. c
5. d
6. d

Describing the Sample
1. Age in years
2. Associate Degree in Nursing
3. 40-49 years

Measures of Central Tendency
1. 3.42
2. 3.10
3. The most frequent score or value that is 3.00 in this example
4. $3.42 + 0.76 = 4.18$ $3.42 - 0.76 = 2.66$
   Range ± 1 *SD* = 2.66 to 4.18 or (2.66, 4.18)

Name That Statistical Test!
1. d   Analysis of variance (ANOVA) testing for group differences with two or more groups; interval or ratio level data
2. a   Chi-square testing for group differences; nominal level data
3. c   Pearson correlation is testing for relationships among variables; interval or ratio level data
4. b   *t*-test testing for differences between two groups; interval or ratio level data

Significance of Results
1. NS
2. *
3. *
4. NS

Crossword Puzzle

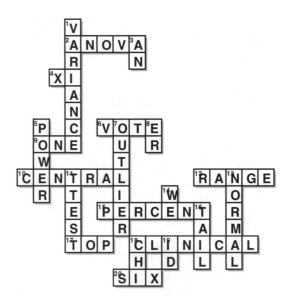

Exercises in Critical Appraisal

Bindler et al. (2007) Study
1. The study had three groups of different ethnic origin: Native American, Hispanic, and Caucasian.
2. Link of variables, level of measurement, and descriptive data analysis techniques

Demographic & Study Variables	Level of Measurement	Descriptive Analysis Techniques
Gender	Nominal	Frequencies, percentages
Age in years	Ratio	Mean, standard deviation, range
Family history of overweight	Nominal	Frequencies, percentages
Systolic blood pressure	Ratio	Mean, standard deviation

3. The mean insulin value in the study was 10.2 μU/ml. The ethnic groups had significantly different insulin values ($p = .043*$) with the Native Americans having the highest insulin value (14.3 μU/ml), the Caucasians were next at 12.0 μU/ml, and the Hispanics had the lowest insulin value (9.2 μU/ml).
4. Regression analysis was used to obtain the results for question 4. The regression model including gender, age, race, body mass index, serum glucose, high-density lipoprotein cholesterol, triglycerides, and blood pressure explained 48% of the insulin level variance.
5. The study limitations included a "small convenience sample that may not be representative of all populations of Native Americans, Hispanic Americans, and Caucasians. In particular, the Native American and Caucasian samples were small. The children were in an agricultural area of central Washington State and may not reflect urban or other diverse populations. Native American tribes and Hispanics from various geographic locations are not uniform in the incidence of type 2 diabetes and risk factors; thus the results cannot be generalized to different tribes or various populations of Hispanics" (p. 211).

Padula et al. (2009) Study
1. Link of variables, level of measurement, and descriptive analysis techniques.

Demographic Variables	Level of Measurement	Descriptive Analysis Techniques
Marital status	Nominal	Frequencies
New York Heart Association Classification	Ordinal	Frequencies
Age in years	Ratio	Mean, range
Mean heart rate	Ratio	Mean

2. The maximal inspiratory pressures (PI_{max}) were significantly different for the treatment group versus the control group. Analysis of variance (ANOVA) was used to obtain this result and the result was $F(3,29) = 8.7$, $p < .0001$.
3. There was no significant difference between the treatment and control groups on physical/functional and psychosocial health-related quality of life (HRQOL) and self-efficacy. The sample size might have been too small to detect differences between the two groups for these psychosocial variables. Thus the study might have had a Type II error of saying there were no significant differences between the two groups when there might have been significance with a larger sample. Also the measurement methods might have some limitations in measuring these study variables. Additional research is needed to determine the impact the inspiratory muscle training (IMT) has on these variables.
4. The researchers clearly identified the clinical applications of their study findings. They indicated that the IMT is a safe and effective intervention to improve inspiratory muscle strength (IMS) in heart failure patients as well as patients with COPD. They also stressed the importance of nurses in supporting and encouraging these patients to keep up their strength.
5. "Recommendations for future research include the following: including subjects with COPD and HF comorbidity as a comparison group because that combination is prominent in this population; tracking the number of doctors' visits and telephone calls preventing emergency room and physician office visits; using a different tool to measure self-efficacy; and evaluating the effects of varying intensity loads. This study has provided evidence that home-based IMT can be effective in improving dyspnea and IMS. However, improvement in QOL and self-efficacy (for breathing) remains questionable. Thus the primary aims were achieved but not the secondary aims; further study is needed" (p. 223).

CHAPTER 12—CRITICAL APPRAISAL OF QUANTITATIVE AND QUALITATIVE RESEARCH FOR NURSING PRACTICE

Key Terms
1. f
2. b
3. a
4. c
5. e
6. d

Key Ideas
1. strengths, weaknesses (limitations), meaning, and significance
2. You might include any three of the following:
   a. What are the major strengths of the study?
   b. What are the major weaknesses or limitations of the study?
   c. Are the findings of the study an accurate reflection of reality?
   d. What is the significance of the findings for nursing?
   e. Are the findings consistent with those of previous studies?
3. You might critically appraise research to share the findings with another health care professional. You might read and critically appraise studies to solve a problem in practice or to summarize research in a topic area for use in practice. You might critically appraise a proposed study to determine whether it is ethical to conduct in your clinical agency.
4. comprehension, comparison, analysis, and evaluation
5. rights, informed consent
6. frame of reference
7. data collection
8. research tradition

Making Connections
1. c
2. b
3. c
4. d
5. a
6. a
7. b
8. d
9. b
10. c

Exercises in Critical Appraisal
Conduct the critical appraisals of the studies included in Appendix B of this study guide. Review the answers to the critical appraisal exercises for Chapters 1 through 11 to assist yourself in these critical appraisals. Also, ask your instructor to clarify any questions that you might have.

CHAPTER 13—BUILDING AN EVIDENCE-BASED NURSING PRACTICE

Key Terms
1. m
2. j
3. i
4. b
5. e
6. g
7. l
8. f
9. d
10. k
11. h
12. c
13. a
14. n

Key Ideas
1. Evidence-based nursing practice promotes desired outcomes for patients, nurses, and health care agencies. You might have identified any of the following reasons for nursing to have evidence-based practice:
   a. Improved quality of care.

    b. Improved patient outcomes such as decreased signs and symptoms, improved functional status, improved physical and psychological health, prevention of illnesses, and increased promotion of health through implementation of healthy lifestyles.

    c. Decreased recovery time.

    d. Decreased need for health care services.

    e. Decreased cost of care.

    f. Improved work environment for nurses with increased productivity.

    g. Increased access to care by providing different types of health care agencies and services with a variety of health care providers.

    h. Increased patient satisfaction with care.

    i. Evidence-based practice important to meet accreditation requirements.

    j. Evidence-based practice is important for a health care agency to achieve magnet status.

2. You might have identified any of the following:

    a. Read research journals in nursing and other health care disciplines.

    b. Read clinical journals with a major focus on publishing research articles.

    c. Use evidence-based websites such as the Agency for Healthcare Research and Quality and many others that communicate evidence-based guidelines and reference a variety of research publications.

    d. Attend professional nursing meetings and conferences.

    e. Attend nursing research conferences.

    f. Participate in collaborative groups of nurses and other health professionals that share research findings.

    g. Note study findings reported on television and on the Internet.

    h. Read research findings reported in newspapers and popular journals.

3. You might have identified any of the following:

    a. Nursing lacks the research evidence in areas for the implementation of evidence-based practice (EBP).

    b. A concern that research evidence generated based on population data might not transfer to the care of individual patients who respond in unique ways.

    c. Best research evidence is currently generated mainly from quantitative and outcomes research methodologies and more work is needed to synthesize qualitative research and determine its contribution to EBP.

    d. EBP movement might lead to the development of evidence-based guidelines that provide a "cookbook" approach to health care.

    e. Health care agencies and administrators do not provide the resources to support the implementation of EBP by nurses.

4. You might have identified any of the following:

    a. EBP requires the synthesis of research evidence from randomized controlled trials and these types of studies are limited in nursing.

    b. Researchers have found limited association between nursing interventions/processes and patient outcomes in acute care settings.

    c. Significant variation in the methods to measure the effect of independent variables (nursing interventions) on patient outcomes.

    d. Need for additional studies to determine the effectiveness of nursing interventions.

    e. Need to identify areas where research evidence is needed for practice.

    f. Nurses need to be more active in conducting quality syntheses (systematic reviews, meta-analyses, and integrative reviews) of research evidence in selected areas.

5. a. Immediate use—using research-based intervention in practice exactly as it was developed.

    b. Reinvention—occurs when the research intervention is modified to meet the needs of a health care agency or nurses within the agency.

    c. Cognitive change—occurs when nurses incorporate research findings into their knowledge bases and use this information to defend a point, write agency protocols or policies, or develop a clinical paper for presentation.

6. a. National Clearinghouse Guideline website (www.guideline.gov) that includes integrative reviews of research. This website was initiated by the Agency for Healthcare Research and Quality.

    b. Cochrane Collaboration that includes systematic reviews, meta-analyses, and integrative reviews of research to determine best research evidence in selected practice areas. The Cochrane Reviews are available at http://www.cochrane.org/reviews/.

    c.   National Library of Health is located in the United Kingdom (UK) and you can search for evidence-based sources using the following website: http://www.evidence.nhs.uk/.

    d.   Meta-analysis—Search CINAHL and MEDLINE for meta-analyses.

    e.   Integrative reviews of research—Search CINAHL and MEDLINE for integrative reviews of research.

7.   The phases of the Stetler Model are:

    a.   Phase I—Preparation

    b.   Phase 11—Validation

    c.   Phase III—Comparative Evaluation/Decision Making

    d.   Phase IV—Translation/Application

    e.   Phase V—Evaluation

8.   Feasibility; current practice

9.   a.   Use research evidence in practice now.

    b.   Consider using research knowledge in practice.

    c.   Do not use the research findings in practice.

10. Iowa

11. Evidence-based guidelines

12. Agency for Healthcare Research and Quality (AHRQ)

13. a.   American Medical Association (AMA)

    b.   American Association of Health Plans (AAHP) now call the American's Health Insurance Plans

14. Evidence-Based Practice Centers

15. Evidence-based practice for nursing

16. the use of research evidence in practice or the use of evidence-based guidelines in practice

Making Connections

Application of the Phases of Stetler's Model

1. a   4. e

2. d   5. b

3. c

Agency's Readiness for Evidence-Based Practice

Obtain the answers to these questions by gathering information in the agency where you are doing your clinical hours this semester. Ask your faculty if these questions might be covered in class.

1.   Review some of the policies in the unit where you are doing clinical and note if the policies are documented with research sources or are the policies without references?

2.   The policies or protocols might be based on the knowledge and experience of the nurses developing them but not documented with research references or evidence-based websites.

3.   Are there nurses in the agency who are responsible for developing and revising policies and procedures and educating nurses to make the necessary changes in practice? Is there a team of nurses working toward meeting accreditation guidelines or magnet status guidelines? These individuals are often the change agents or innovators in an agency.

4.   Ask the staff about access to a library in the agency. Do they have hard copies of journals and what are the names of the journals? Are these research journals or clinical journals with research articles? Do the nurses have access to evidence-based websites on the computers in the agency?

5.   Ask nurses about the goal of evidence-based practice in their agency. What steps have been taken to promote evidence-based practice?

6.   The health care agencies that currently have magnet status can be viewed online at the American Nurses Credentialing Center (ANCC) website at http://www.nursecredentialing.org/Magnet/FindaMagnetFacility.aspx (ANCC, 2009). Look on this website for the status of the agency. If the agency has magnet status, where are they in documenting the outcomes of care to maintain this status? If the agency is seeking magnet status, where are they in the process of obtaining this designation? Having magnet status indicates the agency has a commitment to evidence-based practice.

Exercises in Critical Appraisal

Critical appraisal of the systematic review of childhood obesity prevention developed by Wofford (2008).

1. Was the purpose [or objectives] of the review clearly stated? Provide a rationale.

   Wofford (2008) clearly identified the purpose of the systematic review she conducted. "This systematic review identified the current state of the evidence related to the prevention of obesity in young children" (Wofford, 2008, p. 5).

   "Because there are many published accounts of programs related to obesity prevention with scant or weak evidence, a systematic review of the current literature proved to be helpful in identifying the gaps in the evidence" (Wofford, 2008, p. 6)

2. Did the reviewers report a systematic and comprehensive search strategy to identify relevant studies?

   "The author conducted a systematic and comprehensive literature search using the keywords *child, obesity,* and *prevention.* Search engines used included PubMed, Cochrane Library, Joanna Briggs Institute, and CRISP (Computer Retrieval of Information on Scientific Projects). In addition to these computer-based strategies, hand review of selected bibliography entries was also executed" (Wofford, 2008, p. 6).

3. Were inclusion and exclusion criteria for studies reported and were they appropriate (i.e. was selection bias avoided)?

   "Because the results were voluminous (>5,000 citations), the author limited the fully reviewed articles to those published within the last four years or seminal articles, articles pertaining to preschoolers, articles in the English language, and articles on studies of human subjects" (Wofford, 2008, p. 7). This selection of sources seems appropriate and unbiased.

4. Was the quality of included studies assessed appropriately?

   "Of the many captured articles, 41 were selected for inclusion in the review because of their relevance to the prevention of overweight and obesity in the preschool population and the stronger quality of the evidence they presented. The articles were grouped into five categories. The population-specific group contained five articles, whereas there were seven problem-specific articles. Thirteen articles were included in the guidelines and recommendations groups. The intervention category had 11 articles, and the relevant conceptual models and frameworks section contained five" (Wofford, 2008, p. 7).

5. Were the results of the included studies combined systematically and appropriately?

   The results of the included studies were combined systematically and appropriately as indicated by the following excerpt.

   "During the review of the literature, the author discerned five areas of emphasis—prevalence of the problem, prevention as the best option, preschoolers as the target group, parental involvement as essential, and professional recommendations for interventions. … These grouping threads are important in that they highlight the current state of the literature and provide the reader with an organizing structure to evaluate the evidence. With the use of the organizing structure of five threads or areas of emphasis, gaps were identified and recommendations, which have the potential to direct future research, provide steady foundation for prevention strategies, and encourage increased methodologically rigorous intervention study construction, were proposed" (Wofford, 2008, p. 7). Wofford (2008) also provided tables of the key studies for each of the five threads or areas identified.

6. Were the conclusions supported by the data? (Craig & Smyth, 2007, p. 194)

   The conclusions were clearly stated in the study and seemed supported by the data. "The results indicate five areas of emphasis or threads in the literature: prevalence of the problem; prevention as the best option; preschool population as the target; crucial parental involvement; and numerous guidelines. Because the gap between clear articulation of the problem as well as population and the best strategies to impact the prevention of the problem is evident, health care practitioners must be involved in developing and implementing well-constructed implementation and evaluation studies that build on the limited base of current evidence" (Wofford, 2008, p. 18).

   In summary, Wofford (2008), clearly identified the purpose of her systematic review was to determine the current state of the evidence related to the prevention of obesity in young children. She conducted extensive computer searches of relevant databases and hand reviews of bibliographies to identify relevant sources. Wofford had clearly stated criteria for her selection of the 41 articles that were included in her review. The findings of the review were presented in narrative and studies were summarized in tables related to the five threads: prevalence of the problem, prevention as the best option, preschoolers as the target group, crucial parental involvement, and professional recommendations and guidelines. The studies cited seemed to be of quality and representative of the five threads. The conclusions were reflective of the findings and clearly presented at the end of the article. The author identified what is known and not known about childhood obesity prevention and provided directions for generation of future research evidence, which was the purpose of the review.

Going Beyond
1. Use the content in Chapter 13 to implement an evidence-based practice project guided by Stetler's Model or the Iowa Evidence-based Model.
2. Use the Grove Model to direct the implantation of the evidence-based guidelines.

CHAPTER 14—INTRODUCTION TO OUTCOMES RESEARCH

Key Terms
1. g
2. m
3. h
4. f
5. d
6. l
7. j
8. b
9. e
10. c
11. i
12. a
13. k

Key Ideas
1. the end results of patient care
2. a. The Hospital and Medical Facilities Study Section
   b. The Nursing Study Section
3. Medical Outcomes Study (MOS)
4. a. The effects of nursing interventions on medical outcomes
   b. The effects of staffing patterns on medical outcomes
   c. The effects of nursing practice delivery models on medical outcomes
5. a. Coordination of care
   b. Counseling
   c. Referrals
6. incorporate available evidence on health outcomes into sets of recommendations concerning appropriate management strategies for patients with the studied conditions
7. inclusion of nursing data in the large databases used to analyze outcomes
8. outcome
9. a. Clinical guidelines
   b. Critical paths
   c. Care maps
10. Large heterogeneous
11. a. Information about the patient, such as disease severity, comorbidity, and types of outcomes
    b. Processes of care provided
    c. Patient status over time
    d. Follow-up information
12. You might have listed any of the following questions:
    a. What proportion of people experiencing a specific cluster of symptoms were diagnosed (correctly or not) as having a particular condition?
    b. Who received what treatment?
    c. Should a treatment or procedure have been performed?
    d. Did persons with a particular diagnosis receive the appropriate treatment?
    e. What proportion of people with the cluster of symptoms receive no treatment?
    f. Was the treatment effective?
13. a. There is no clearly superior treatment for all individuals with a given problem.
    b. There are a number of treatments with some proven efficacy that are relatively comparable in their effectiveness in undifferentiated groups of subjects.
    c. There is evidence of differential outcome either within or across treatments for defined subtypes of clients.

14. most consistent with nursing theory and practice
15. change across time for the study subjects
16. American Nurses Association
17. a. Mean improvement score for all patients treated
    b. The percentage of patients who improved
    c. Whether all patients improved slightly or whether there is a divergence among patients; with some improving greatly, whereas others do not improve at all
    d. Characteristics of patients who experience varying degrees of improvement
    e. Characteristics of outliers
18. You might identify any two of the following:
    a. The North American Nursing Diagnosis Association (NANDA) Classification
    b. The Omaha System
    c. The Home Health Care Classification
    d. The Nursing Intervention Classification (NIC); also, the Nursing Outcomes Classification (NOC)
19. percentage
20. dissemination of findings

Making Connections

Research Strategies for Outcomes Studies

1. e
2. c
3. g
4. f
5. a
6. d
7. b

Major Contributors to Outcomes Research
1. d: U.S. government agency that promotes nursing research
2. c: Data are collected regarding benchmarking data
3. b: National professional nursing organization
4. a: Agency developed from Agency for Health Care Policy and Research to promote the conduct, synthesis, and use of research findings in practice
5. e: Classification system that includes nursing interventions

Exercises in Critical Appraisal
Critically appraise the Kanak, Titler, Shever, Fei, Dochterman, & Picone (2008) article found in the 'Research Articles' section of the Evolve resources for Understanding Nursing Research *at http://evolve.elsevier.com/burns/understanding.*
1. Kanak et al. (2008) article is an outcomes study as indicated by the study purpose and design.
2. The outcomes being considered by this study are expressed in the study purpose and research questions: "The purpose of this study was to describe the impact of multiunit hospitalizations on selected nursing treatments, resource use, and clinical outcomes. After controlling for the primary medical diagnosis, severity of illness, and comorbid medical conditions, three research questions were addressed:
    1. What is the effect of a patient residing on multiple inpatient units during a hospitalization on the average daily use of the nursing treatments of patient teaching and discharge planning?
    2. What is the effect of a patient residing on multiple inpatient units during a hospitalization on resource use (length of stay, total hospital cost)?
    3. What is the effect of a patient residing on multiple inpatient units during a hospitalization on the clinical outcomes of nosocomial infection, adverse occurrence, patient fall, medication error, discharge disposition, and mortality?" (Kanak et al., 2008, p. 16)
3. The data and sample for this study were extracted from a large data repository of a primary study on nursing outcomes effectiveness research.
4. The findings of the study are: "A significant association was found between hospitalizations on multiple units and selected nursing treatments, resource use, and all clinical outcomes except for mortality. Nurses play a central role in coordinating the care that patients receive across inpatient units and are positioned to develop and implement strategies to mediate the negative impacts associated with patients moving across multiple units" (Kanak et al., 2008, p. 15).

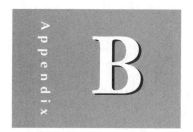

B Published Studies

Metabolic Syndrome in a Multiethnic Sample of School Children: Implications for the Pediatric Nurse

Ruth C. McGillis Bindler, RNC, PhD
Linda K. Massey, RD, PhD
Jill Armstrong Shultz, PhD
Paulette E. Mills, PhD
Robert Short, PhD

There is lack of translational work that may assist the pediatric nurse in identifying the child who is at risk for metabolic syndrome. Early identification of the syndrome could assist pediatric health care providers in intervening and in lowering child health risks. Fasting serum insulin, metabolic syndrome criteria, and dietary intake were examined in a multiethnic sample of children aged 9–15 years. Forty-seven percent had two or more risk factors for metabolic syndrome, and 28% had three or more risk factors. Insulin levels were negatively correlated with the recommended dietary allowance. A regression model, including gender, age, race, body mass index, serum glucose, high-density lipoprotein cholesterol, triglycerides, and blood pressure, explained 48% of insulin variance.
© 2007 Elsevier Inc. All rights reserved.

METABOLIC SYNDROME, ALSO known as dysmetabolic syndrome, syndrome X, or insulin resistance syndrome, is characterized by a group of risk factors and is often a precursor to both diabetes and cardiovascular disease. These risk factors cluster in individuals and populations, both in adults and in youths. The syndrome is typified by a decrease in the number of insulin receptors and in their functional ability at the cellular level (insulin resistance), with resultant hyperinsulinemia and development of type 2 diabetes as the pancreas attempts to compensate. The United States Cholesterol Education Program Adult Treatment Panel III (ATP III) recommended the diagnosis of metabolic syndrome in adults when three of five symptoms are found: high triglyceride levels, low high-density lipoprotein cholesterol (HDL-C), hypertension, obesity (particularly with central adiposity), and fasting glucose > 6.1 mmol/l (110 mg/dl) (National Institutes of Health, 2001). These criteria reflect the major metabolic components of the syndrome, which are abdominal obesity, atherogenic dyslipidemia, increased blood pressure (BP), insulin resistance, proinflammatory state, and prothrombotic state (Grundy, Brewer, Cleeman, Smith, & Lenfant, 2004). Other groups have recommended somewhat different criteria, leading to confusion among clinicians (see Table 1 for a summary of adult criteria recommendations for metabolic syndrome) (Zimmet, Magliano, Matsuzawa, Alberti, & Shaw, 2005).

REVIEW OF LITERATURE

One in four Americans is at risk for developing metabolic syndrome (Ford, Giles, & Dietz, 2002; Roberts, Dunn, Jean, & Lardinois, 2000). Life-

From the Intercollegiate College of Nursing, Washington State University, Spokane, WA, Food Science and Human Nutrition Department, Washington State University, Spokane, WA, Food Science and Human Nutrition Department, Washington State University, Pullman, WA, Human Development Department, Washington State University, Pullman, WA, and Biostatistics, The Washington Institute, Washington State University, Spokane, WA.

Address correspondence and reprint requests to Ruth C. McGillis Bindler, RNC, PhD, Intercollegiate College of Nursing, Washington State University, West 2917 Fort George Wright Drive, Spokane, WA 99224-5291. E-mails: bindler@wsu.edu, massey@wsu.edu, armstroj@wsu.edu, pmills@wsu.edu, rshort@wsu.edu

0882-5963/$ - see front matter
© 2007 Elsevier Inc. All rights reserved.
doi:10.1016/j.pedn.2006.05.008

Table 1. Criteria for Metabolic Syndrome, Used in Adults

World Health Organization	ATP III	International Diabetes Federation
Diabetes mellitus, impaired glucose tolerance, or inclusion in the top quartile of fasting insulin (if nondiabetic), plus two or more of following:	Three or more of following:	Waist circumference > 102 cm for males or > 88 cm for females (or ethnic-specific values), plus two or more of following:
BMI > 30	Waist circumference > 102 cm for males or > 88 cm for females	Triglycerides > 150 mg/dl (1.7 mmol/l) or treatment for this condition
Triglycerides ≥ 150 mg/dl (1.7 mmol/l) or HDL-C < 35 mg/dl (0.9 mmol/l)	Triglycerides > 150 mg/dl (1.7 mmol/l)	HDL-C < 40 mg/dl (1.03 mmol/l) for males or < 50 mg/dl (1.29 mmol/l) for females, or treatment for this condition
BP ≥ 140/90 mm Hg or on medication	HDL-C < 40 mg/dl (1.03 mmol/l) for males or < 50 mg/dl (1.29 mmol/l) for females	BP > 130/85 mm Hg or on medication
Albumin ≥ 20 µg/min or albumin:creatinine ratio ≥ 30 mg/g	BP > 130/85 mm Hg or on medication	Fasting plasma glucose ≥ 100 mg/dl (5.6 mmol/l) or diagnosed type 2 diabetes mellitus
	Fasting plasma glucose > 110 mg/dl (6.1 mmol/l)	

Note: Data from Zimmet et al. (2005).

style, environment, and genetic component are influential in the syndrome. Lifestyle factors that contribute to the problem are high-saturated-fat and low-fiber diets, stress, and lack of physical activity (Kelley, 2000; Ludwig et al., 1999; Mayer-Davis et al., 1997). The environment promotes metabolic syndrome when there is limited opportunity for daily physical activity or limited access to fresh and nutritious food choices. Lifestyle and environmental factors are closely related, but both may play independent and interactive parts in the emergence of metabolic syndrome. Genetic factors place certain population groups, such as Native Americans and Hispanic Americans, at higher risk for diabetes and insulin resistance (Cruz et al., 2004; Valdez, 2000).

Due to an epidemic in youth obesity and sedentary behaviors, there is an increasing need to describe the factors associated with the development of insulin resistance in youths. For children, only one risk factor, in addition to being overweight, has been suggested as adequate reason to screen for additional clinical abnormalities (Falkner, Hassink, Ross, & Gidding, 2002). Although there is no clear consensus on the criteria for metabolic syndrome in children, on the number of criteria needed for diagnosis, or on the differences in criteria at various ages, some researchers have adapted adult metabolic syndrome criteria to the examination of child data. For example, in one analysis, the criteria used to define adolescent metabolic syndrome included fasting triglycerides ≥

110 mg/dl; HDL-C ≤ 40 mg/dl; fasting glucose ≥ 110 mg/dl; abdominal measurement ≥ 90th percentile for age and gender; and BP ≥ 90th percentile for age, gender, and height (Cook, Weitzman, Auinger, Nguyen, & Dietz, 2003). Another group of researchers defined adolescent metabolic syndrome when three or more of the following criteria were met: fasting triglycerides ≥ 1.1 mmol/l (100 mg/dl); HDL-C < 1.2 mmol/l (45 mg/dl) for male adolescents 15–19 years old and 1.3 mmol/l (50 mg/dl) for all others; fasting glucose > 6.1 mmol/l (110 mg/dl); waist circumference > 75th percentile for age and gender; and systolic BP > 90th percentile for gender, age, and height (de Ferranti et al., 2004). Others have used similar criteria, with differences, including: triglycerides ≥ 90th percentile for age and gender; HDL-C < 10th percentile for age and gender; and impaired glucose tolerance identified by a glucose level of 140–200 mg/dl following a 2-hour postchallenge glucose test (Cruz et al., 2004; Shaibi et al., 2005). Still another group of researchers has used a body mass index (BMI) *z* score ≥2.0; fasting glucose > 140 mg/dl (7.8 mmol/l); triglycerides > 95th percentile; HDL < 5th percentile; and BP > 95th percentile for age and gender (Weiss et al., 2004). Age ranges vary in the studies; thus, no findings and age-specific criteria have been developed. It has been noted that there is as yet no agreement about the criteria for the overall assessment and treatment of metabolic syndrome in children and adolescents (Golley, Magarey,

Table 2. Criteria for Metabolic Syndrome, Used in Children

Criteria	Data from Cook et al. (2003)	Data from de Ferranti et al. (2004)	Data from Cruz et al. (2004)	Data from Weiss et al. (2004)	Present Study
Triglycerides	≥ 110 mg/dl (1.24 mmol/l)	≥ 100 mg/dl (1.1 mmol/l)	≥ 90th percentile	> 95th percentile	≥ 110 mg/dl (1.24 mmol/l)
HDL-C	≤ 40 mg/dl (1.03 mmol/l)	< 45 mg/dl (1.2 mmol/l) for males 15–19 years and < 50 mg/dl (1.3 mmol/l) for all others	< 10th percentile	< 5th percentile	≤ 40 mg/dl (1.03 mmol/l)
Glucose	≥ 110 mg/dl (6.1 mmol/l) for fasting level	> 110 mg/dl (6.1 mmol/l) for fasting level	140–200 mg/dl (7.8–11.1 mmol/l) following a 2-hour postchallenge glucose test	> 140 mg/dl (7.8 mmol/l) for fasting level	≥ 110 mg/dl (6.1 mmol/l) for fasting level
Adiposity	≥ 90th percentile for abdominal measurement	> 75th percentile for abdominal measurement	≥ 90th percentile for abdominal measurement	BMI z-score ≥ 2.0	≥ 85th percentile for BMI
BP	≥ 90th percentile	≥ 90th percentile	≥ 90th percentile	≥ 95th percentile	≥ 90th percentile

Steinbeck, Baur, & Daniels, 2006; Steinberger & Daniels, 2003) (see Table 2 for a summary of metabolic syndrome criteria for childhood, as applied by various researchers).

Although it is unclear exactly which criteria should be used to identify metabolic syndrome in children and adolescents, a rapid rise in the prevalence of obesity, abdominal girth, and type 2 diabetes in youths necessitates attention to the issue. One study applied the same 1999–2000 criteria for metabolic syndrome (those described in Cook et al., 2003) to the National Health and Nutrition Examination Survey (NHANES) data for 1988–1992 and found that the rate of the syndrome, defined by the presence of three criteria, increased from 4.2% to 6.4% in that short span of years (Duncan, Li, & Zhou, 2004). The increase in obesity and type 2 diabetes creates the urgent need for research that will assist in the establishment of universal criteria for metabolic syndrome in children (Molnar, 2004). Pediatric nurses are often unfamiliar with metabolic syndrome and need solid research and evidence-based recommendations to apply what is known about this condition to their work with children in a variety of settings.

Few studies have described metabolic syndrome or the marker of insulin in children, and even fewer have examined childhood ethnic differences in risks. A clustering of syndrome variables in children, including high serum triglycerides, low HDL-C, and high glucose, adiposity, and high BP, was found to explain 55% of serum insulin variance (Srinivasan, Myers, & Berenson, 1999). Impaired fasting glucose and type 2 diabetes have

been identified in children using data from national health surveys (Fagot-Campagna, Saaddine, Flegal, & Beckles, 2001). Insulin was an independent predictor of triglycerides in obese children (Valle et al., 2002).

Most research studies on ethnic variations and metabolic syndrome have included only Black and White children. The Bogalusa Heart Study has studied Black and White children, noting the persistence of elevated insulin levels from childhood into adulthood in all children (Bao, Srinivasan, & Berenson, 1996; Chen et al., 2000), higher triglyceride and insulin levels in Black children than in White children (Chen, Srinivasan, Elkasabany, & Berenson, 1999), and higher dyslipidemia and higher insulin secretion in White obese adolescents than in Black obese adolescents, with low insulin sensitivity in both groups (Bacha, Saad, Gungor, Janosky, & Arslanian, 2003). In other studies, Black children showed greater insulin resistance than White children, even after adjustment for body composition, social class, and dietary intake patterns (Lindquist, Gower, & Goran, 2000). Furthermore, obesity, greater visceral fat, and Black ethnicity were identified as negative and independent health risks (Gower, Nagy, & Goran, 1999). The incidence of hyperinsulinemia in a sample of overweight Black and White 11- to 18-year-olds was 30%; hyperinsulinemic children had significantly higher BMI, total cholesterol (TC), low-density lipoprotein (LDL), triglycerides, glucose, and insulin:glucose ratio (Sullivan et al., 2004).

Native American/Alaskan Native/First Nation and Hispanic children are at-risk ethnic groups needing further delineation of factors related to metabolic syndrome. Although there are a limited number of studies focusing on ethnic minority groups, the data available demonstrate an increased incidence of risk factors in these groups. In Canadian First Nation children, fasting insulin and glucose levels were associated with BMI percentile (Young, Dean, Flett, & Wood-Steinman, 2000). An analysis of studies on type 2 diabetes in children reported that disease incidence among North American Indians varied from 2.3/1,000 for Canadian Cree and Ojibway to 4.5/1,000 for all U.S. American Indians, to 50.9/1,000 for Pima Indians in the southwest United States (Fagot-Campagna et al., 2000). In one analysis of health records in Montana and Wyoming Indian Health Service facilities, > 50% of cases of diabetes in youths were type 2 (Harwell et al., 2001).

Hispanic children have a higher incidence of overweight and hypertension than White, Black, and Asian children (Sorof, Lai, Turner, Poffenbarger, & Portman, 2004). In addition, the prevalence of impaired glucose tolerance (a precursor to metabolic syndrome and type 2 diabetes) was 17.8% among Hispanic adolescents, as compared with 7% in all ethnic groups (Williams et al., 2002). Although Hispanics in the United States come from many different countries and may have different risk factors, a major group originated from Mexico, and several studies have been carried out with Hispanics of Mexican origin. Mexican American children have a high rate of obesity (27% for female children and 23% for male children) (Suminski, Poston, & Foreyt, 1999), and 45% of new cases of diabetes in Mexican American youths are type 2 (Neufeld, Raffel, Landon, Dhen, & Vadheim, 1998). Analysis of NHANES data for 1999–2000 demonstrates the increasing problem of overweight in Mexican American children because 22.7% of 2- to 5-year-olds, 39.3% of 6- to 11-year-olds, and 43.8% of 12- to 19-year-olds were overweight or were at risk for overweight (Ogden, Flegal, Carroll, & Johnson, 2002). Mexican American adults 20 years and older demonstrate a higher incidence of metabolic syndrome (31.9%) than Whites (23.8%) (Ford et al., 2002).

Many of the criteria for metabolic syndrome are related to dietary intake, and ethnicity may play a part in food choices. High levels of dietary fat intake have been identified in Black youth as compared with other ethnic groups (Lindquist et al.,

2000; Weigensberg et al., 2005). However, in a study comparing the dietary intake of White and Native American children in Oklahoma, a high rate of low-nutrient-dense and high-fat foods was ingested by both groups with no significant differences by ethnicity (Stroehla, Malcoe, & Velie, 2005). A study of Hispanic and non-Hispanic toddlers found that intakes at meals and snacks were not significantly different between the two groups (Ziegler, Hanson, Ponza, Novak, & Hendricks, 2006).

Children, in general, and those from Native American and Hispanic groups, in particular, are underrepresented in diabetes and cardiovascular disease origins research. There is scant application of identification methods for metabolic syndrome in the nursing literature. More information is needed to establish the contribution of various characteristics to insulin resistance in children, and translational research is needed so that findings can be applied by nurses and other health professionals in pediatric settings. Descriptive data about children, particularly from disparate ethnic groups, will help to identify children at highest risk so that appropriate interventions can be identified. Clear guidelines for nurses will assist in applying findings about metabolic syndrome to pediatric settings with youths.

PURPOSE

The purpose of this study was to describe serum insulin levels and to investigate their relationships to metabolic syndrome criteria in a multiethnic sample of school children. Furthermore, analysis of results of dietary recall with the criteria for metabolic syndrome was performed to draw conclusions about the usefulness of dietary intake history. Descriptive data, including demographics, physical measurements, dietary intakes, and physical activity characteristics, were analyzed for within-group differences. Specific assessments and referral criteria for nursing practice were developed using the results. The specific research questions were as follows:

1. What are the fasting serum insulin levels in a multiethnic sample of school children in central Washington State?
2. What are the relationships between insulin levels and the criteria for metabolic syndrome in a multiethnic sample of children in central

Washington State? See operational definition of metabolic syndrome criteria below.

3. What are the relationships between reported dietary intake and metabolic syndrome criteria?
4. Which data predict insulin levels in this multiethnic sample of children?
5. How can the information learned in this study be used by pediatric nurses in clinical settings?

Operational Definitions

1. In this study, the criteria for metabolic syndrome were selected from those most often used in other studies. These include the following:

a. High triglycerides, ≥ 1.24 mmol/l (110 mg/dl)
b. Low HDL-C, ≤ 1.03 mmol/l (40 mg/dl)
c. Hypertension, $\geq$ 90th percentile considering age, gender, and height percentile
d. Overweight, $\geq$ 85th percentile BMI considering age, gender, height, and weight
e. Elevated fasting glucose, ≥ 6.1 mmol/l (110 mg/dl)
f. Elevated fasting insulin, ≥ 15 μU/ml

2. Borderline high fasting insulin, ≥ 15–20 μU/ml; high fasting insulin, > 20 μU/ml.

METHODS

Sample

The convenience sample consisted of 100 children (representing approximately 15% of eligible students) attending fourth to eighth grades at public elementary and middle schools in a predominantly agricultural area of central Washington State. Parents received a flyer about the study (written in English and Spanish languages), which was sent home from school through the children. They could elect to attend an informational program (conducted in both English and Spanish languages) in school one evening. If they signed a consent, their children were informed about the study and could choose whether to sign an assent and participate. Only children with no identified illnesses or medications were included because blood draws and exercise tests were to be performed. Participants who spoke English or Spanish were eligible. Children could select a small gift from a basket at the end of data collection. The protocol was approved by the Institutional Review Boards

of Spokane, Washington, and Washington State University, and the school board of the district where the study was conducted.

Procedures and Instruments

Study personnel consisted of a registered nurse/ nutrition doctoral student, eight baccalaureate nursing students, a phlebotomist, one dietitian, and one dietetics student. All were trained and evaluated for reliability on measurement and for assistance to children during questionnaire completion. All measurements and questionnaires involving the children were implemented within a single day in the children's schools. Data were collected in large rooms at the schools and separated into stations for testing. The phlebotomist completed serum venous blood draws on the children. The children's body measurements, BP, and exercise tests were completed by the nurse and nursing students. All diet recalls and questionnaires were completed with the children by the dietitian and by the dietetics student.

Parents of children in the study completed a medical family history form (accomplished during the informational evening session, or accomplished and sent later) developed by the Make Early Diagnoses–Prevent Early Deaths Program at the University of Utah. This questionnaire asked about early cardiovascular disease, diabetes, overweight, and hypertension among parents, siblings, grandparents, aunts, and uncles of the children. Parents were also asked to identify to which ethnic groups their children belonged. All forms were available in English and Spanish languages.

Blood draws were completed in the early morning by the licensed phlebotomist after the children had fasted for at least 10 hours; children were then fed breakfast before completing the remainder of the testing. Fasting blood samples were tested for glucose, TC, HDL-C, and triglycerides using the Beckman CX 5Delta analyzer, and low-density lipoprotein cholesterol (LDL-C) was calculated by applying the Friedewald equation [(TC − HDL-C) − triglycerides / 5]. Insulin was measured by solid-phase radioimmunoassay with the Coat-A-Count Insulin System (Diagnostic Products, Los Angeles, CA).

The smoking history of the children was collected on a questionnaire that asked if they were current smokers or if they had ever tried smoking. BP was measured on the right arm at heart level while the children were sitting; three readings were made with a 5-minute rest in between, and the mean of the three readings was used in the analysis. Percentile analysis was performed using grids from the National Heart, Lung, and Blood Institute (2004) that take into account height percentile, age, and gender. Metabolic-cost-of-activity (MET) scores were calculated from the children's reported history of weekly physical activity on the Godin Leisure Time Questionnaire (Godin & Shephard, 1985; Kriska & Casperson, 1997). Physical measurements of height, weight, triceps skinfold thickness, and the Canadian Aerobic Fitness Test (to calculate VO_{2max}) were obtained in uniform and recommended ways. BMI was calculated as weight: height ratio (kg/m^2); percentiles for height, weight, triceps skinfold, and BMI were obtained from the National Center for Health Statistics growth grids (Centers for Disease Control and Prevention, 2000). Because no measure of central adiposity was completed, BMI $\geq$ 85th percentile was used as the obesity criterion for metabolic syndrome in this sample.

Dietary data were collected by the use of the Youth/Adolescent Question (YAQ) (Rockett et al., 1997; Rockett & Colditz, 1997). This 151-item food frequency questionnaire has been used with children from 8 to 18 years and correlates well (0.54) with 24-hour diet recall results. It uses the Statistical Analysis System and calculates means and standard deviations for energy and all nutrients. It collects data about the intake of food items for days, weeks, and months. The trained nursing students and the dietitian assisted subjects, as needed, with the questionnaire and had a list of foods common to Hispanic and Native American communities to add, as necessary, to individual child forms. Completed questionnaires were returned to YAQ developers at the Harvard School of Public Health for the calculation of the dietary intake of nutrients from the questionnaire and for the calculation of the percentage of recommended dietary allowance (RDA) for each nutrient.

In addition, a 24-hour diet recall was completed verbally with each child by a trained dietitian. These results were used to calculate Healthy Eating Index (HEI) scores. The HEI was designed by the United States Department of Agriculture to measure how the diets of Americans conform to dietary guidelines. It provides a score from 0 = *low* to 10 = *high* for 10 components of the diet. Each of the scores is then added for a composite score, with a total possible score of 100. The 10 HEI scores are for grains, vegetables, fruit, milk, meat, total fat,

saturated fat, cholesterol, sodium, and variety (Bowman, Lino, Gerrior, & Basiotis, 1998; Kennedy, Ohls, Carlson, & Fleming, 1995; Variyam, Smallwood, & Basiotis, 1998).

Statistical Analysis

Statistical analyses were carried out using the Statistical Package for the Social Sciences (SPSS), version 12.0. Each variable was examined for skewness, and the mean and standard deviation were described. Chi-square test was used to test categorical data, and one-way analysis of variance was used to test continuous variables. The probability levels of .05 and .01 were considered significant and highly significant, respectively. Kendall's τ was used to assess correlations between variables. Stepwise linear regression was used to explore the variables that were influential in explaining insulin variance. An odds ratio for meeting at least three risk criteria on the dichotomized insulin variable was computed using binary logistic regression.

RESULTS

Description of the Sample

The age range of the sample was 9–15 years (M = 12 years). The sample included 52 boys and 48 girls. Sixty-four (64%) claimed to be purely Hispanic, 15 (15%) claimed to be purely Native American, and 9 (9%) claimed to be purely Caucasian. Twelve (12%) additional subjects claimed to have mixed-race ethnic heritage. All Hispanic children had Mexico as origin of the family and were employed in farming or food processing industries. There were no significant differences among ethnic groups regarding age or gender; reported family history of cardiovascular disease, diabetes, overweight, or smoking; physical activity; weight percentiles; BMI percentiles; or triceps skinfold percentiles. Table 3 shows the demographic data and physical measurements of the total sample and of the ethnic subsample (those children identifying with just one major ethnic group). Blood samples were not obtained on two children; thus, serum analysis was completed on 98 children. The 98 children who had blood drawn are included in this analysis (referred to as the total sample); when race differences are examined, calculations are reported on the 86 children who listed just one ethnic group in their demographic profile and had a successful

Table 3. Demographics and Physical Measures, by Ethnic Group

Variables	Total Sample (N = 100)	Ethnic Subsample (n = 88)	Native American (n = 15)	Hispanic (n = 64)	Caucasian (n = 9)	p
Gender						
Male	52 (52%)	43 (49%)	7 (47%)	30 (47%)	6 (67%)	.529
Female	48 (48%)	45 (51%)	8 (53%)	34 (53%)	3 (33%)	
Age (years)	11.8 ± 1.6	11.9 ± 1.5	12.4 ± 1.6	11.9 ± 1.5	11.3 ± 1.5	.183
Range	9–15	9–15	9–14	9–15	9–13	
Family history						
Cardiovascular disease	52 (52%)	42 (48%)	5 (33%)	31 (48%)	6 (67%)	.279
Diabetes	28 (28%)	24 (27%)	4 (27%)	19 (30%)	1 (11%)	.503
Overweight	53 (53%)	43 (49%)	6 (40%)	32 (50%)	5 (56%)	.717
Smoking	74 (74%)	63 (72%)	11 (73%)	43 (67%)	9 (100%)	.122
Physical activity						
VO_{2max}						.506
< Avg	35 (35%)	30 (34%)	6 (40%)	20 (31%)	4 (44%)	
Avg	32 (32%)	29 (33%)	3 (20%)	22 (34%)	4 (44%)	
> Avg	33 (33%)	29 (33%)	6 (40%)	22 (34%)	1 (11%)	
MET score (Avg)	57 ± 25.0	56.0 ± 25.0	52.2 ± 24.3	54.3 ± 23.8	73.8 ± 30.4	.074
Smoking history (+)	20 (20%)	17 (19.3%)	8 (53%)	8 (13%)	1 (11%)	.001**
x̄ Systolic BP (mm Hg)	109.2 ± 9.8	109.4 ± 10.0	112.6 ± 10.2	107.7 ± 9.6	116.4 ± 8.8	.017*
x̄ Diastolic BP (mm Hg)	68.7 ± 11.6	68.8 ± 12.2	73.1 ± 9.3	66.8 ± 12.6	75.4 ± 9.7	.040*
x̄ Height percentile	58.4 ± 29.5	57 ± 30	55 ± 29	54 ± 30	81 ± 15	.035*
x̄ Weight percentile	71.1 ± 29.2	70 ± 30	82 ± 25	65 ± 31	81 ± 26	.074
x̄ BMI percentile	75.6 ± 25.2	74 ± 26	84 ± 27	72 ± 26	75 ± 27	.283
x̄ Skinfold percentile	66.0 ± 28.7	65 ± 30	78 ± 28	62 ± 29	62 ± 38	.169

Notes: Statistics are frequencies (%) and means ± standard deviations. p is from one-way analysis of variance. Avg = average.

*Significant at the .05 level (two-tailed test).

**Significant at the .01 level (two-tailed test).

serum blood draw (referred to as ethnic subsample). Further characteristics of the study participants have been previously described (Bindler, Massey, Shultz, Mills, & Short, 2004).

There was a highly significant difference among ethnic groups regarding child smoking history, with a higher frequency of "having tried smoking" reported by Native American children. Significant differences in mean systolic BP and mean diastolic BP were found, with Caucasians having the highest pressures (116/75 mm Hg), followed by Native Americans (113/73 mm Hg), and with Hispanics having the lowest BPs (108/67 mm Hg). Although there were no group differences for weight and BMI percentiles, there was a significant difference among the groups in mean height percentile, with the Caucasians being taller (M = 81st percentile) than either the Native American group (M = 55th percentile) or the Hispanic group (M = 54th percentile). Dietary analysis showed no significant differences among ethnic groups in terms of carbohydrate, protein, fat, calorie, sucrose, or fiber intakes. Likewise, there were no differences among groups in the percentage of calories from fat and the kilocalories of intake per kilogram of weight (Table 4).

The mean fasting glucose was 4.75 mmol/l (85.8 mg/dl), and all but four children had a value below 5.5 mmol/l (100 mg/dl), with no significant differences among ethnic groups. Those with serum glucose above 5.5 mmol/l had values

ranging from 5.66 to 6.00 mmol/l. No children had glucose above 6.1 mmol/l (110 mg/dl).

Research Question 1: What Are the Fasting Serum Insulin Levels in a Multiethnic Sample of School Children in Central Washington State?

The mean insulin value was 10.2 µU/ml, with significant differences found among ethnic groups (Native Americans > Caucasians > Hispanics). Eighty percent (n = 78) had normal insulin levels (< 15 µU/l), whereas 7% (n = 7) had borderline high levels (15–20 µU/l) and 13% (n = 13) had high levels (> 20 µU/l).

Research Question 2: What Are the Relationships Between Insulin Levels and the Criteria for Metabolic Syndrome in a Multiethnic Sample of Children in Central Washington State?

Fifty-one children (51%) had BMI ≥ 85th percentile; 20 (20%) had triglycerides above 1.24 mmol/l (110 mg/dl); 24 (24%) had HDL-C ≤ 1.03 mmol/l (40 mg/dl); 14 (14%) had systolic BP ≥ 90th percentile; 24 (24%) had diastolic BP ≥ 90th percentile; and 31 (31%) had either systolic BP or diastolic BP ≥ 90th percentile for height, age, and gender.

Only two children in this convenience sample had no risk factors for metabolic syndrome. Forty-seven (47%) had two factors, 28 (28%) had three

Table 4. Mean Serum Measures and Dietary Intake, by Ethnic Group

Variables	Total Sample	Ethnic Subsample	Subgroups			p
			Native American	Hispanic	Caucasian	
Serum	N = 98	N = 86	N = 15	N = 62	N = 9	
TC (mmol/l)	4.30 ± 0.64	4.28 ± 0.66	4.25 ± 0.60	4.31 ± 0.68	4.09 ± 0.65	.626
LDL-C (mmol/l)	2.60 ± 0.58	2.60 ± 0.60	2.43 ± 0.61	2.64 ± 0.57	2.52 ± 0.67	.462
HDL-C (mmol/l)	1.27 ± 0.26	1.25 ± 0.27	1.33 ± 0.29	1.25 ± 0.26	1.17 ± 0.31	.391
Triglycerides (mmol/l)	0.93 ± 0.56	0.94 ± 0.57	1.07 ± 0.60	0.92 ± 0.59	0.85 ± 0.40	.617
Glucose (mmol/l)	4.75 ± 0.44	4.76 ± 0.45	4.87 ± 0.55	4.73 ± 0.45	4.82 ± 0.21	.530
Insulin (µU/ml)	10.2 ± 7.2	10.3 ± 7.28	14.3 ± 9.9	9.2 ± 5.7	12.0 ± 10.4	.043*
Dietary	N = 100	N = 88	N = 15	N = 64	N = 9	
Carbohydrate (g)	313.9 ± 236.4	308.0 ± 235.6	235.4 ± 359.1	335.2 ± 208.8	234.7 ± 112.6	.208
Protein (g)	80.1 ± 56.5	78.2 ± 53.9	78.3 ± 86.9	79.1 ± 47.1	71.0 ± 28.3	.916
Total fat (g)	79.3 ± 56.0	78.3 ± 55.6	75.2 ± 83.5	79.6 ± 50.9	73.5 ± 30.5	.929
Saturated fat (g)	28.4 ± 19.0	28.1 ± 18.8	26.4 ± 25.7	28.4 ± 17.9	28.6 ± 12.3	.929
Polyunsaturated fat (g)	14.4 ± 11.3	14.3 ± 11.4	13.6 ± 17.4	14.7 ± 10.3	12.6 ± 6.4	.846
Calories from fat (%)	31.1 ± 5.4	31 ± 6.0	31 ± 6.2	31 ± 5.0	37 ± 6.1	.876
Calories (kcal)	2,306 ± 1,565	2,218 ± 2,350	2,218 ± 2,351	2,343 ± 1,398	1,859 ± 786	.141
Calories/weight (kcal/kg)	50.1 ± 38.7	41.5 ± 46.7	41.5 ± 46.7	52.8 ± 38.8	38.1 ± 18.1	.111
Sucrose (g)	67.5 ± 47.6	68.0 ± 48.2	63.7 ± 65.6	72.3 ± 45.9	44.6 ± 21.0	.257
Fiber (g)	19.1 ± 14.1	18.5 ± 13.5	18.2 ± 19.0	19.5 ± 12.4	12.4 ± 9.2	.342

*Significant at the .05 level (two-tailed test).

Table 5. Incidence of Risk Factors for Metabolic Syndrome

Risk Factors	Native American	Hispanic	Caucasian	Mixed Race
BP > 90th percentile	5 {33%} {n = 15}	21 {33%} {n = 64}	4 {44%} {n = 9}	1 {8%} {n = 12}
BMI > 85th percentile	10 {67%} {n = 15}	29 {45%} {n = 64}	5 {56%} {n = 9}	7 {58%} {n = 12}
Triglycerides ≥ 110 mg/dl	3 {20%} {n = 14}	13 {20%} {n = 63}	2 {22%} {n = 9}	2 {17%} {n = 12}
HDL < 40 mg/dl	1 {7%} {n = 14}	15 {24%} {n = 63}	3 {33%} {n = 9}	1 {8%} {n = 12}
Glucose > 100 mg/dl	0	0	0	

Note: Variation in *n* among variables reflects two children from whom blood could not be obtained.

factors, and 4 (4%) had four metabolic syndrome factors. The most common risk factor displayed was increased BMI percentile, with high BP being the next most common factor shown (Table 5).

Significant positive relationships were found between insulin and increasing age ($F = 6.164$, $p = .015$, $df = 1,79$), between insulin and female gender ($F = 3.972, p = .050, df = 1,79$), and between insulin and Native American race ($F = 3.372$, $p = .039$, $df = 2,79$). Female Native American children had the highest mean insulin levels (17.9 μU/ml), whereas Hispanic male children had the lowest mean values (6.6 μU/ml) (Figure 1). Although 6 of 9 (67%) Caucasian children and 54 of 63 (86%) Hispanic children had normal insulin levels, only 8 of 14 (57%) Native American children had normal insulin values. All of the Native American children with elevated insulin levels were in the highest category (> 20 μU/l).

Insulin showed highly significant positive correlations with systolic and diastolic BP; weight, BMI, and skinfold percentiles; serum triglycerides and glucose; and triglyceride:HDL and TC:HDL ratios. Furthermore, insulin showed significant

positive correlations with having tried smoking, height percentile, and serum TC and LDL-C. It had highly significant negative correlations with total dietary fat and kilocalories per kilogram of weight. It had significant negative correlations with dietary carbohydrate, protein, total calories, percentage of calories from fat, and serum HDL-C (Table 6). Insulin resistance index (IRI) was calculated using the model fasting insulin (μU/ml) × fasting glucose (mmol/l) / 22.5. Because the relational statistics for IRI as the outcome variable were nearly the same as those using insulin as the outcome variable, only the findings using insulin are reported.

Research Question 3: What Are the Relationships Between Reported Dietary Intake and Metabolic Syndrome Criteria?

The results of both the HEI obtained by an analysis of 24-hour diet recalls and the

Glucose mean = 85.8 mg/dl
Insulin mean = 10.3 μU/ml (range 2–32)

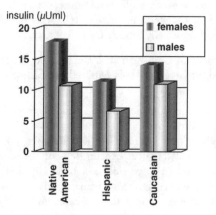

Figure 1.   Serum insulin levels, by ethnic group and gender.

Table 6. Correlates of Insulin

Variables	Kendall's τ	ρ
Age	.265**	.001
Sex	−.306**	.001
Family history		
Cardiovascular disease	.129	.149
Diabetes	.128	.153
Overweight	−.045	.613
VO$_{2max}$	−.016	.852
MET score	−.027	.720
Smoking history	.206*	.021
Systolic BP	.345**	< .001
Diastolic BP	.311**	< .001
Height percentile	.198*	.012
Weight percentile	.396**	< .001
BMI percentile	.399**	< .001
Skinfold percentile	.392**	< .001
Serum		
TC	.157*	.034
LDL-C	.163*	.028
HDL-C	−.216**	.004
Triglycerides	.303**	.001
Glucose	.246**	.007

*Correlation is significant at the .05 level.
**Correlation is significant at the .01 level.

Table 7. Dietary Correlates of Metabolic Syndrome Criteria

Variables	Systolic BP > 90th Percentile	Diastolic BP > 90th Percentile	BMI (%)	Glucose	HDL	Triglycerides	Insulin
HEI Grains	−.084	−.071	−.116	−.012	.022	.043	.021
HEI Veggies	−.083	.007	−.070	.052	−.014	.040	.037
HEI Fruit	−.090	.071	−.075	−.009	−.036	.073	.072
HEI Milk	.070	−.078	−.057	−.021	−.103	−.025	−.098
HEI Meat	.066	.007	−.017	.047	−.024	−.004	.050
HEI Fat	−.089	.112	−.002	−.163*	−.069	.168*	−.051
HEI SatFat	−.063	.059	.049	−.062	.015	.200**	.019
HEI Chol	.035	.201*	.017	−.012	.012	.182*	−.048
HEI Sod	−.023	−.012	0.61	−.074	−.005	−.057	−.082
HEI Var	−.148	−.034	−.067	−.037	.099	−.100	−.065
HEI Total	−.065	.088	−.026	−.064	−.055	.164*	−.019
Calories	−.169*	−.192*	−.153*	−.060	.105	−.130	−.209**
Protein	−.152	−.172	−.139	−.045	.139*	−.161*	−.226**
Carbs	−.166*	−.226	−.149*	−.071	.084	−.088	−.197**
Cal/kg	−.256**	−.263**	−.351**	−.103	.197**	−.203**	−.360**
Fat	−.165*	−.173*	−.187**	−.018	.156*	−.200**	−.253**
SatFat	−.131	−.154	−.182*	.009	.126	−.194**	−.223**
MonoFat	−.172*	−.176*	−.183*	−.025	.169*	−.218**	−.258**
PolyFat	−.165*	−.170*	−.158*	−.018	.155*	−.188**	−.270**
Omega 3	−.172*	−.203*	−.149*	−.005	.266**	−.153*	−.215**
Chol	−.179*	−.188*	−.156*	−.008	.133	−.185**	−.236**
Fiber	−.129	−.132	−.072	−.026	.087	−.064	−.026
Ca (% RDA)	−.057	−.104	−.059	.017	.070	−.081	−.146*
Fe (% RDA)	−.129	−.132	−.072	−.064	.108	−.088	−.233**
Vitamin C (% RDA)	−.072	−.133	−.060	−.014	.064	−.039	−.129
Vitamin B1 (% RDA)	−.106	−.109	−.087	−.038	.072	−.076	−.186**
Vitamin B2 (% RDA)	−.103	−.126	−.071	−.030	.094	−.086	−.165*
Niacin (% RDA)	−.147	−.093	−.103	−.079	.101	−.108	−.209**
Vitamin B6 (% RDA)	−.117	−.121	−.050	−.040	.070	−.081	−.187**
Folate (% RDA)	−.106	−.091	−.053	−.029	.028	−.048	−.143*
Vitamin B12 (% RDA)	−.106	−.101	−.033	.084	.147*	−.109	−.145*
Vitamin A (% RDA)	−.041	−.109	.066	.015	.006	.037	−.071
Vitamin D (% RDA)	.014	−.115	−.043	.050	.091	−.069	−.160*
Vitamin E (% RDA)	−.105	−.049	−.049	.044	.047	−.042	−.152*

*Correlation is significant at the .05 level.
**Correlation is significant at the .01 level.

dietary nutrient intakes obtained by a food frequency questionnaire were examined by correlations with the risk factors for metabolic syndrome (Table 7). There were two major findings from this analysis.

First, there were many significant negative relationships between serum insulin and the percentage of RDA for nutrients, suggesting that when dietary recalls identify several nutrients not ingested at the recommended level, children may be at risk for insulin resistance and metabolic syndrome.

Second, a lower fat intake of the recommended types of fats, such as monounsaturated, polyunsaturated, and omega 3 fatty acids, is related to a higher incidence of metabolic risk. The reason for several negative correlations between

the reported intake of calories per kilogram and the incidence of metabolic syndrome criteria is unclear and may relate to the lack of reliability of dietary recall, especially among child reporters.

Research Question 4: Which Data Predict Insulin Levels in This Multiethnic Sample of Children?

A regression model that included gender, age, race, BMI percentile, serum glucose, HDL-C, triglycerides, systolic BP, and diastolic BP was tested and found to explain 48% of the variance in insulin. Triglycerides, systolic BP, and race were removed in a backward stepwise procedure, with the resulting model explaining 50% of insulin variance (Table 8). Using binary logistic stepwise regression, the odds ratio for having

Table 8. Linear Regression of Insulin With Metabolic Syndrome Variables

Variables	β Coefficient	t	p
Regression I			
Gender	−3.535	−3.010	.004
Age	.983	2.434	.017
Race	−.586	−.494	.622
BMI percentile	9.409E−02	3.368	.001
Glucose	.275	3.480	.001
Triglycerides	5.566E−03	.409	.684
HDL-C	−.137	−2.136	.036
Systolic BP	−4.493E−02	−4.68	.641
Diastolic BP	.109	1.543	.127
Adjusted R^2 = .484, $p \le$ .001			
Regression II			
Gender	−3.702	−3.270	.002
Age	1.039	2.699	.009
BMI percentile	9.415E−02	3.810	.000
Glucose	.258	3.570	.001
HDL-C	−.137	−2.382	.020
Diastolic BP	8.808E−02	1.596	.115
Adjusted R^2 = .499, $p \le$ .001			

elevated insulin was 5.8 (95% confidence interval = 1.5–22.1) when three or more risk factors were present.

DISCUSSION

In this study, the most commonly used criteria were adapted from adults and from various recommendations for the application of criteria to child populations. Insulin levels in this study showed large variability, and 20% of children had borderline or high insulin levels. Consistent with other studies, insulin levels showed a positive correlation with criteria for metabolic syndrome, including high BP, high adiposity (measured in this study by BMI percentiles), high serum triglycerides and glucose, and low serum HDL-C. The odds ratio of having elevated insulin when three risk criteria were present was nearly six times that seen in children without this combination of risk factors.

Total carbohydrate, protein, and fat intake showed negative associations with insulin, as did kilocalories consumed per kilogram. The latter factor was not correlated with MET scores or VO_{2max}—the two measures of physical activity used. These findings were unexpected. Intake and insulin levels, particularly at kilocalories per kilogram, would be expected to show positive correlations. Perhaps the diet recalls did not accurately reflect dietary intake for the children—a common problem with this method of nutritional

analysis. Negative correlations between RDAs for many nutrients and serum insulin levels suggested that diet histories can be used to identify children with aberrant insulin levels. Interventions to target RDAs are appropriate to improve the general dietary and metabolic profile.

Although fiber intake was not a significant correlate with insulin, its levels and trends were in the direction expected. Children at the ages used in the study should have a daily dietary fiber intake of 26 g (female children) to 38 g (male children) (Food and Nutrition Board, 2002); the mean for this sample was 19.1 g. A pattern of low fiber, high fat, and total energy intake in insulin resistance, along with characteristic lipid profiles, has been identified by researchers working with young adults (Ludwig et al., 1999; Van Horn, 1997).

Although the criteria for metabolic syndrome were demonstrated across ethnic groups in this study, the risk of the syndrome appeared to be highest in the Native American female children in the sample. It was notable that the Native American children had the highest BMI percentiles—a measure of adiposity. Regression analysis found that race was not a significant factor in insulin variance, but that BMI percentile was highly significant. In addition, mean skinfold percentile, another measure of adiposity, was high among the Native American group. This is consistent with the Bogalusa Heart Study findings that obesity was linked to the development of hyperinsulinemia (Srinivasan et al., 1999) and with studies linking childhood obesity to insulin resistance syndrome (Weiss et al., 2004). Perhaps high weight and BMI percentiles in Native Americans in this study, in comparison with their more average height percentiles, place them at greater risk for insulin resistance. However, the food frequency questionnaire did not identify a total caloric intake greater than those in the other ethnic groups studied.

Another factor of potential importance is that about half of the Native American children had tried smoking. Although not directly associated with insulin resistance, if this behavior persists into adulthood, it is clearly an additional risk in both diabetes and cardiovascular disease. One study has found a positive association of metabolic syndrome criteria with tobacco exposure and serum cotinine levels in adolescents (Weitzman et al., 2006).

It would have been expected that the Hispanic sample subjects would have a high incidence of elevated insulin and would display a high risk of metabolic syndrome. This was not the case, perhaps because the study was performed in a farming area where many from among the Hispanic population were migrant workers who had not lived in the United States for long. In addition, the town was small and had only one fastfood restaurant. Eating out was not a common occurrence for most migrant families. This demonstrated that ethnic variations found in other studies should be explored within specific communities. Assumptions should not be made about a particular sample or population based on national findings or on the results of other studies in diverse geographic areas. Such considerations are important in light of findings that racial and ethnic minorities tend to receive a lower quality of health care than nonminorities and that differences in certain disease risk may be present (National Academy of Sciences, 2002).

The present study had several limitations. The sample was a small convenience sample and may not be representative of all populations of Native Americans, Hispanic Americans, and Caucasians. In particular, the Native American and Caucasian samples were small. The children were in an agricultural area of central Washington State and may not reflect urban or other diverse populations. Native American tribes and Hispanics from various geographic locations are not uniform in the incidence of type 2 diabetes and in risk factors; thus, the results cannot be generalized to different tribes or various populations of Hispanics. In spite of being a convenience sample, finding no significant differences among group members in the intake of essential nutrients supports the representativeness of the sample. Future studies may lead to enhanced knowledge by adding measures of central adiposity and puberty staging to collection procedures.

CLINICAL IMPLICATIONS

A major problem in the application of research on metabolic syndrome by nurses in various settings is the lack of a clear definition of criteria that signify the syndrome. A variety of cutoff points for criteria, such as serum triglycerides, HDL-C, and glucose, has been used both in adults (Table 1) and in children (Table 2). When considering children, the use of different definitions for metabolic syndrome leads to confusion. For example, in a study that contrasted the prevalence of metabolic syndrome in 1,513 Black,

White, and Hispanic adolescents using World Health Organization versus U.S. National Cholesterol Education Program ATP III definitions, the incidence was 8.4% versus 4.2%, respectively, when using the different criteria (Goodman, Daniels, Morrison, Huang, & Dolan, 2004). In a study of 99 children, the percentage of children diagnosed with metabolic syndrome varied from 0–4% to 39–60%, depending on which set of six criteria was used (Golley et al., 2006). Nurses in schools, offices, and other settings are justifiably confused about which children should be identified as at-risk and in need of further referral.

Research Question 5: How Can the Information Learned in This Study Be Used by Pediatric Nurses in Clinical Settings?

Although specific guidelines to identify insulin resistance in children are not available, some information is clear and application to clinical settings is possible. The clustering of variables seen in many children makes identification of metabolic syndrome easier in clinical situations. Several criteria of the syndrome are routinely measured in child health care visits. This study demonstrated that evaluation of common data such as BMI and BP provides critical information, and it therefore supports the recommendations of other pediatric nurses (Hardy, Harrell, & Bell, 2004; Yensel, Preud'Homme, & Curry, 2004). Height, weight, BMI, and BP are commonly assessed, but careful analysis of results is not always performed. BMI and BP must be measured on each child, and percentiles must be determined. This practice can be integrated into all child health care settings, such as clinics, schools, well-child visits, episodic illness care, and hospitalization.

Information gained from BMI and BP can be expanded on in at-risk children by referring them for the measurement of serum lipids, glucose, and insulin. Triglycerides, HDL-C, and glucose results should be examined where they have been obtained, such as in office or clinic settings. When this total profile is available, an abnormality in three of five assessment criteria (BMI, BP, triglycerides, HDL-C, and glucose) necessitates referral for further data gathering and intervention. In addition, the nurse should be alert to a family history of cardiovascular disease and diabetes, and for membership in high-risk ethnic groups such as Native Americans/Alaskan Natives, Hispanics, and Pacific Islanders. These may be considered additional risk factors, especially when serum levels of lipids and glucose are not available.

Dietary analysis is a supplementary tool that can be used by pediatric nurses in some settings. Although there may not be time to complete recalls in all situations, it may be possible to have families write down the child's 24-hour intake, do a quick check or analyze the diet, and contact the family later with specific suggestions. The child who does not meet a variety of RDAs should be targeted for dietary teaching, particularly if BMI and BP also show abnormalities.

Diabetes and cardiovascular disease pose continuing public health problems for our population and, in particular, for the minority groups represented in this study. The rates of type 2 diabetes have risen, particularly in the ethnic groups studied here and among children. Although glucose levels are commonly believed to be definitive for diabetes, they may not indicate a prediabetes or an insulin-resistant state. A key finding of this study is that, even when fasting glucose levels are normal, insulin may be increased and can indicate a pattern of insulin resistance. Furthermore, baseline insulin in childhood has been linked to hypertriglyceridemia at 6-year follow-up (Raitakari et al., 1995). The presence of three or more metabolic syndrome risk factor criteria in this study was highly suggestive of elevated insulin

and may guide nurses and other care providers in clinical settings to establish a definitive set of interventions designed to lower risk in these children, even when serum insulin levels are not available (see Table 9).

SUMMARY

In summary, this study found significant correlations of insulin with body adiposity, BP, and serum lipid/lipoprotein levels, consistent with the clustering of variables labeled as metabolic syndrome. Furthermore, there were ethnic and gender differences in serum insulin levels, indicating an increased risk of metabolic syndrome among Native Americans, particularly among Native American female children, as compared to Hispanic and Caucasian populations. Research efforts need to confirm these findings with larger groups and with Native American tribes and Hispanic samples in a variety of geographic locations. Longitudinal studies would help to demonstrate the persistence of syndrome variables over time with individual children and populations, further guiding intervention efforts. In addition, higher insulin levels were related to a lower incidence of meeting the RDAs for dietary nutrients. Future research is needed to provide clear guidelines for the identification of insulin resistance and metabolic syndrome in youths to design interventions that decrease the incidence of type 2 diabetes and the emergence of cardiovascular disease (Cruz & Goran, 2004). At this time, it is known that overweight is a critical risk factor that is associated with insulin resistance, dyslipidemia, and BP elevations (Steinberger, 2003). Therefore, nurses must be certain that height and weight are measured on all children and that the results are analyzed for BMI and placed on appropriate growth charts. Accurate BP measurement is needed, with the use of grids for analysis, to determine those above the 90th and 95th percentiles. Weight elevations should signal the need for careful further assessment for other risk factors, such as family history, smoking, failure to meet RDAs in dietary intake, physical inactivity, abnormal lipid levels, and, in some cases, abnormal glucose and insulin levels. Pediatric nurses are critically important in the early identification of a cascade of health risk factors, which begins with overweight, continues through elevated BP and other characteristics, and

---

Table 9. Measures to Identify Children at Risk for Metabolic Syndrome

Schools, clinics, and other community settings

1. Measure height and weight. Compute percentiles. Compute BMI and BMI percentile. Consider children at ≥ 85th percentile to be at risk and children at ≥ 95th percentile to be at high risk.
2. Measure BP. Use charts to evaluate percentile. Consider children at ≥ 90th percentile to be at risk and children at ≥ 95th percentile to be at high risk.
3. Complete dietary recall and analyze diet for deficiencies and excesses. Consider that multiple differences from RDAs may be indicative of abnormal insulin levels.
4. Consider family history of diabetes, overweight, hypertension, and cardiovascular disease as risk factors.
5. Refer to health care provider for additional assessment when more than one risk is observed.
6. Intervene to improve diet and physical activity for children with risks. Provide family and child with resources to lower risks.

Pediatric offices

1. When the child is overweight and has another risk factor, recommend fasting serum analysis for glucose and lipids/lipoproteins.
2. Plan an intervention program to lower the risks identified. Reevaluate the child's risk at least annually.

becomes metabolic syndrome and, subsequently, type 2 diabetes.

ACKNOWLEDGMENTS

The support of the Society for Pediatric Nurses, the Delta Chi Chapter-at-Large of Sigma Theta Tau International, the Intercollegiate College of Nursing/Washington State University College of Nursing Carl M. Hansen Research Fund, the Glen King Fellowship in Nutrition at the Washington State University, The Heart Institute of Spokane, and the Westcoast Hospitality is gratefully acknowledged.

REFERENCES

Bacha, F., Saad, R., Gungor, N., Janosky, J., & Arslanian, S. A. (2003). Obesity, regional fat distribution, and syndrome X in obese black versus white adolescents: Race differential in diabetogenic and atherogenic risk factors. *The Journal of Clinical Endocrinology and Metabolism, 88,* 2534–2540.

Bao, W., Srinivasan, S. R., & Berenson, G. S. (1996). Persistent elevation of plasma insulin levels is associated with increased cardiovascular risk in children and young adults. *Circulation, 93,* 54–59.

Bindler, R. C., Massey, L. K., Shultz, J. A., Mills, P. E., & Short, R. (2004). Homocysteine in a multi-ethnic sample of school-age children. *Journal of Pediatric Endocrinology and Metabolism, 17,* 327–337.

Bowman, S. A., Lino, M., Gerrior, S. A., & Basiotis, P. P. (1998). The health eating index: 1994–1996. Washington, DC: U.S. Department of Agriculture, Center for Nutrition Policy and Promotion CNPP-5.

Centers for Disease Control and Prevention. (2000). CDC growth charts: United States. Available from http://www.cdc.gov/growthcharts/.

Chen, W., Bao, W., Begum, S., Elkasabany, A., Srinivasan, S. R., & Berenson, G. S. (2000). Age-related patterns of the clustering of cardiovascular risk variables of syndrome X from childhood to young adulthood in a population made up of black and white subjects. The Bogalusa Heart Study. *Diabetes, 49,* 1042–1048.

Chen, W., Srinivasan, S. R., Elkasabany, A., & Berenson, G. S. (1999). Cardiovascular risk factors clustering features of insulin resistance syndrome (syndrome X) in a biracial (black–white) population of children, adolescents, and young adults. *American Journal of Epidemiology, 150,* 667–674.

Cook, S., Weitzman, M., Auinger, P., Nguyen, M., & Dietz, W. H. (2003). Prevalence of a metabolic syndrome phenotype in adolescents. *Archives of Pediatric and Adolescent Medicine, 157,* 821–827.

Cruz, M. L., & Goran, M. I. (2004). The metabolic syndrome in children and adolescents. *Current Diabetes Reports, 4,* 53–62.

Cruz, M. L., Weigensberg, M. J., Huang, T. T. K., Ball, G., Shabi, G. Q., & Goran, J. I. (2004). The metabolic syndrome in overweight Hispanic youth and the role of insulin sensitivity. *Journal of Clinical Endocrinology and Metabolism, 89,* 108–113.

de Ferranti, S. D., Gauvreau, K., Ludwig, D. S., Neufeld, E. J., Newburger, J. W., & Rifai, N. (2004). Prevalence of the metabolic syndrome in American adolescents: Findings for the Third National Health and Nutrition Examination Survey. *Circulation, 110,* 2494–2497.

Duncan, G. E., Li, S. J., & Zhou, X. H. (2004). Prevalence and trends of a metabolic syndrome phenotype among U.S. adolescents, 1999–2000. *Diabetes Care, 27,* 2438–2443.

Fagot-Campagna, A., Pettitt, D. J., Engelgau, M. M., Burrows, N. R., Geiss, L. S., Valdez, R., et al. (2000). Type 2 diabetes among North American children and adolescents: An epidemiologic review and a public health perspective. *Journal of Pediatrics, 136,* 664–672.

Fagot-Campagna, A., Saaddine, J. B., Flegal, K. M., & Beckles, G. L. A. (2001). Diabetes, impaired fasting glucose, and elevated HbA_{1c} in U.S. adolescents: The Third National Health and Nutrition Examination Survey. *Diabetes Care, 24,* 834–837.

Falkner, B., Hassink, S., Ross, J., & Gidding, S. (2002). Dysmetabolic syndrome: Multiple risk factors for premature adult disease in an adolescent girl. *Pediatrics, 110,* e 14 [Retrieved from http://pediatrics.aappublications.org/cgi/content/full/110/1/e14].

Food and Nutrition Board, Institute of Medicine. (2002). Dietary reference intakes for energy, carbohydrates, fiber, fat, fatty acids, cholesterol, protein, and amino acids (macronutrients). Washington, DC: National Academy Press.

Ford, E. S., Giles, W. H., & Dietz, W. H. (2002). Prevalence of the metabolic syndrome among US adults: Findings from the Third National Health and Nutrition Examination Survey. *The Journal of the American Medical Association, 287,* 356–359.

Godin, G., & Shephard, R. J. (1985). A simple method to assess exercise behavior in the community. *Canadian Journal of Applied Sports Science, 10,* 141–146.

Golley, R. K., Magarey, A. M., Steinbeck, K. S., Baur, L. A., & Daniels, L. A. (2006). Comparison of metabolic syndrome prevalence using six different definitions in overweight pre-pubertal children enrolled in a weight management study. *International Journal of Obesity, 30,* 853–860.

Goodman, E., Daniels, S. R., Morrison, J. A., Huang, B., & Dolan, L. M. (2004). Contrasting prevalence of and demographic disparities in the World Health Organization and National Cholesterol Education Program Adult Treatment Panel III definitions of metabolic syndrome among adolescents. *Journal of Pediatrics, 145,* 445–451.

Gower, B. A., Nagy, T. R., & Goran, M. I. (1999). Visceral fat, insulin sensitivity, and lipids in prepubertal children. *Diabetes, 48,* 1515–1521.

Grundy, S. M., Brewer, H. B., Cleeman, J. I., Smith, S. C., & Lenfant, C. (2004). Definition of metabolic syndrome: Report of the National Heart, Lung, and Blood Institute/American Heart Association conference on scientific issues related to definition. *Circulation, 109,* 433–438.

Hardy, L. R., Harrell, J. S., & Bell, R. A. (2004). Overweight in children: Definitions, measurements, confounding factors, and health consequences. *Journal of Pediatric Nursing, 19,* 376–384.

Harwell, T. S., McDowall, J. M., Moore, K., Fagot-Campagna, A., Helgerson, S. D., & Gohdes, D. (2001).

Establishing surveillance for diabetes in American Indian youth. *Diabetes Care, 24,* 1029–1032.

Kelley, D. E. (2000). Overview: What is insulin resistance? *Nutrition Reviews, 58,* S2-S3.

Kennedy, E. T., Ohls, J., Carlson, S., & Fleming, K. (1995). The healthy eating index: Design and applications. *Journal of the American Dietetic Association, 95,* 1103–1111.

Kriska, A. M., & Casperson, C. J. (1997). Introduction to a collection of physical activity questionnaires. *Journal of the American College of Sports Medicine 29,* S5–S9, S36-S38.

Lindquist, C. H., Gower, B. A., & Goran, M. I. (2000). Role of dietary factors in ethnic differences in early risk of cardiovascular disease and type 2 diabetes. *American Journal of Clinical Nutrition, 71,* 725–732.

Ludwig, D. S., M. A.Pereira, D. S., Kroenke, C. H., Hilner, J. E., Van Horn, L., Slattery, M. L., et al. (1999). Dietary fiber, weight gain, and cardiovascular disease risk factors in young adults. *The Journal of the American Medical Association, 282,* 1539–1546.

Mayer-Davis, E. J., Monaco, J. H., Hoesn, H. M., Carmichael, S., Vitolins, M. Z., & Rewers, M. J. (1997). Dietary fat and insulin sensitivity in a triethnic population: The role of obesity. The Insulin Resistance Atherosclerosis Study (IRAS). *American Journal of Clinical Nutrition, 65,* 79–87.

Molnar, K. (2004). The prevalence of the metabolic syndrome and type 2 diabetes in children and adolescents. *International Journal of Obesity, 28,* S70-S74.

National Academy of Sciences. (2002). Unequal treatment: Confronting racial and ethnic disparities in health care. Retrieved from http://www.nap.eduopenbook/030908265X.html.

National Heart, Lung, and Blood Institute. (2004). Fourth report on the diagnosis, evaluation and treatment of high blood pressure in children and adolescents. Retrieved from http://www.nhlbi.gov/guidelines/hypertension/child_tbl.htm.

National Institutes of Health. (2001). Third report of the National Cholesterol Education Program Expert Panel on detection, evaluation and treatment of high blood cholesterol in adults. Bethesda, MD: National Institutes of Health [NIH Publication 01-3670].

Neufeld, N. D., Raffel, L. J., Landon, C., Dhen, Y. D., & Vadheim, C. M. (1998). Early presentation of type 2 diabetes in Mexican–American youth. *Diabetes Care, 21,* 80–86.

Ogden, C. L., Flegal, K. M., Carroll, M. D., & Johnson, C. L. (2002). Prevalence and trends in overweight among US children and adolescents. *The Journal of the American Medical Association, 288,* 1728–1732.

Raitakari, O. T., Porkka, K. V. K., Ronnemaa, T., Knip, M., Uhari, M., Akerblom, H. K., et al. (1995). The role of insulin in clustering of serum lipids and blood pressure in children and adolescents: The Cardiovascular Risk in Young Finns Study. *Diabetologia, 38,* 1042–1050.

Roberts, K., Dunn, K., Jean, S. K., & Lardinois, C. K. (2000). Syndrome X: Medical nutrition therapy. *Nutrition Reviews, 58,* 154–160.

Rockett, H. R. H., Breitenbach, M., Frazier, A. L., Witschi, J., Wolf, A. M., Field, A. E., et al. (1997). Validation of a youth/adolescent food frequency questionnaire. *Preventive Medicine, 26,* 808–816.

Rockett, H. R. H., & Colditz, G. A. (1997). Assessing diets of children and adolescents. *American Journal of Clinical Nutrition Supplement, 65,* 1116S–1122S.

Shaibi, G. Q., Cruz, M. L., Ball, G. D., Weigensberg, M. J., Kobaissi, H. A., Salem, G. J., et al. (2005). Cardiovascular

fitness and the metabolic syndrome in overweight Latino youths. *Medicine and Science in Sports and Exercise, 37,* 922–928.

Sorof, J. M., Lai, D., Turner, J., Poffenbarger, T., & Portman, R. J. (2004). Overweight, ethnicity, and the prevalence of hypertension in school-aged children. *Pediatrics, 113,* 475–482.

Srinivasan, S. R., Myers, L., & Berenson, G. S. (1999). Temporal association between obesity and hyperinsulinemia in children, adolescents and young adults: The Bogalusa Heart Study. *Metabolism, 48,* 928–934.

Steinberger, J. (2003). Diagnosis of the metabolic syndrome in children. *Current Opinion in Lipidology, 14,* 555–559.

Steinberger, J., & Daniels, S. R. (2003). Obesity, insulin resistance, diabetes, and cardiovascular risk in children. An American Heart Association Scientific Statement from the Atherosclerosis, Hypertension, and Obesity in the Young Committee (Council on Cardiovascular Disease in the Young) and the Diabetes Committee (Council on Nutrition, Physical Activity, and Metabolism). *Circulation, 107,* 1448–1453.

Stroehla, B. C., Malcoe, L. H., & Velie, E. M. (2005). Dietary sources of nutrients among rural Native American and white children. *Journal of the American Dietetic Association, 105,* 1908–1916.

Sullivan, C. S., Beste, J., Cummings, D. M., Hester, V. H., Holbrook, T., Kolasa, K. M., et al. (2004). Prevalence of hyperinsulinemia and clinical correlates in overweight children referred for lifestyle intervention. *Journal of the American Dietetic Association, 104,* 433–436.

Suminski, R. R., Poston, W. S., & Foreyt, J. P. (1999). Early identification of Mexican American children who are at risk for becoming obese. *International Journal of Obesity, 23,* 823–829.

Valdez, R. (2000). Epidemiology. *Nutrition Reviews, 58,* S4-S6.

Valle, M., Gascon, F., Martos, R., Ruz, F. J., Bermudo, F., Morales, R., et al. (2002). Metabolic cardiovascular syndrome in obese prepubertal children: The role of high fasting insulin levels. *Metabolism, 51,* 423–428.

Van Horn, L. (1997). Fiber, lipids, and coronary heart disease. *Circulation, 95,* 2701–2704.

Variyam, J. B., Smallwood, C., & Basiotis, P. P. (1998). USDA's healthy eating index and nutrition information. Washington, DC: USDA Center for Nutrition Policy and Promotion [Technical Bulletin No. 1866].

Weigensberg, M. J., Ball, G. D., Shaibi, G. Q., Cruz, M. L., Gower, B. A., & Goran, M. I. (2005). Dietary fat intake and insulin resistance in black and white children. *Obesity Research, 13,* 1630–1637.

Weiss, R., Dziura, J., Burgert, T. S., Tamborlane, W. V., Taksali, S. E., Yeckel, C. W., et al. (2004). Obesity and the metabolic syndrome in children and adolescents. *New England Journal of Medicine, 350,* 2362–2374.

Weitzman, M., Cook, S., Auinger, P., Florin, T. A., Daniels, S., Nguyen, M., et al. (2006). Tobacco smoke exposure is associated with the metabolic syndrome in adolescents. *Circulation, 112,* 862–869.

Williams, C. L., Hayman, L. L., Daniels, S. R., Robinson, T. N., Steinberger, J., Paridon, S., et al. (2002). Cardiovascular health in childhood: A statement for health professional from the Committee on Atherosclerosis, Hypertension, and Obesity in the Young (AHOY) of the Council on Cardiovascular Disease in the Young, American Heart Association. *Circulation, 106,* 143–160.

Yensel, C. S., Preud'Homme, D., & Curry, D. M. (2004). Childhood obesity and insulin-resistant syndrome. *Journal of Pediatric Nursing, 19,* 238–246.

Young, T. K., Dean, H. J., Flett, B., & Wood-Steinman, P. (2000). Childhood obesity in a population at high risk for type 2 diabetes. *Journal of Pediatrics, 136,* 365–369.

Ziegler, P., Hanson, C., Ponza, M., Novak, T., & Hendricks, K. (2006). Feeding infants and toddler study: Meal and snack intakes of Hispanic and non-Hispanic infants and toddlers. *Journal of the American Dietetic Association, 106,* 107–123.

Zimmet, P., Magliano, D., Matsuzawa, Y., Alberti, G., & Shaw, J. (2005). The metabolic syndrome: A global public health problem and a new definition. *Journal of Atherosclerosis and Thrombosis, 12,* 295–300.

Available online at www.sciencedirect.cor

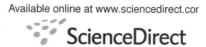

ScienceDirect

Applied Nursing Research 22 (2009) 18–25

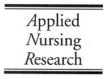

Applied
Nursing
Research

www.elsevier.com/locate/apnr

A home-based nurse-coached inspiratory muscle training intervention in heart failure

Cynthia A. Padula, PhD, RN, CS[a],*, Evelyn Yeaw, PhD, RN[a], Saurabh Mistry, MS[b]

[a]*College of Nursing, University of Rhode Island, Kingston, RI 02881, USA*
[b]*College of Pharmacy, University of Rhode Island, Kingston, RI 02881, USA*

Received 10 September 2006; revised 20 February 2007; accepted 22 February 2007

Abstract

People with heart failure (HF) are living longer but with disabling dyspnea that erodes quality of life (QOL). Decreased strength of inspiratory muscles (IMs) may contribute to dyspnea in HF, and inspiratory muscle training (IMT) has been shown to improve the strength of IMs. The purpose of this study was to determine the effects of a 3-month nurse-coached IMT program. Bandura's Self-Efficacy Theory directed nursing interventions. This randomized controlled trial employed an experimental group (IMT) and a control group (education). Data were collected during six home visits. Outcome measures included maximal inspiratory pressure, perceived dyspnea, self-efficacy, and health-related QOL. Significant differences in PI_{max}, dyspnea, and respiratory rate were found. Implications for further research and practice are discussed.
© 2009 Elsevier Inc. All rights reserved.

1. Introduction

Heart failure (HF) is a major public health problem affecting more than 5 million people in the United States and is the leading cause of repeat hospitalizations (American Heart Association, 2000). People with HF are living longer but with disabling symptoms, particularly dyspnea, that erode quality of life (QOL) (American Heart Association, 2000). Decreased strength of inspiratory muscles (IMs) may contribute to the dyspnea in HF (Vibarel et al., 2002). Inspiratory muscle training (IMT) has been shown to increase the performance of IMs in patients with chronic obstructive pulmonary disease (COPD) (Larson, Covey, & Corbridge, 2002). COPD and chronic HF are diseases with similar muscular problems, including the mechanisms and clinical impact of muscle dysfunction (Caroci & Lareau, 2004). The goal of this study was to determine the effect of IMT on people with HF. It was hypothesized that IMT would increase the strength of IMs, decrease dyspnea, and have a positive effect on health-related QOL (HRQOL).

2. Literature review

2.1. Dyspnea in chronic HF

Dyspnea is a complex multifaceted sensation influenced by a variety of factors (Larson et al., 2002). Dyspnea associated with HF has traditionally been explained by hemodynamic and neurohormonal models (Gibbs, Keegan, Wright, Fox, & Poole-Wilson, 1990), but these do not adequately explain the breathlessness associated with chronic HF (Rogers, 2001). The muscle hypothesis (Clark, Poole-Wilson, & Coats, 1996), which suggests abnormalities of skeletal muscle as the source of symptoms, must be considered. Skeletal muscle function and bulk are reduced in HF and contribute to symptoms (McConnell, Mandak, Sykes, Fesniak, & Dasgupta, 2003). Respiratory and skeletal muscle changes, resulting from disease and inactivity, cause increased ventilation at rest and with exercise, contributing to breathlessness (McConnell et al., 2003). In HF, impaired IMs result in reductions in strength, endurance, and functional performance (Vibarel et al., 2002).

2.2. IMT: Overview

Respiratory muscle strength and endurance can be increased with IMT, given adequate training load (Larson

* Corresponding author. Tel.: +1 401 874 5344; fax: +1 401 874 5346.
  E-mail addresses: cpadula@cox.net (C.A. Padula),
eyeaw@cox.net (E. Yeaw).

0897-1897/$ – see front matter © 2009 Elsevier Inc. All rights reserved.
doi:10.1016/j.apnr.2007.02.002

C.A. Padula et al. / Applied Nursing Research 22 (2009) 18–25　　　　　　19

et al., 2002); inspiratory threshold loading represents the most widely used method. Maximal inspiratory pressure (PI_{max}) and maximal expiratory pressure (PE_{max}) reflect the combined strength of respiratory muscles (Larson & Kim, 1987). The training device is a clear plastic cylinder with an inscribed scale of centimeters of water pressure, an airflow valve at one end, and an internal pressure regulator that can be easily adjusted by turning a plastic rod. The subject breathes through a mouthpiece with a nose clip in place, generating pressure to open the airflow valve. The study of IMT in COPD has spanned more than two decades; more recently, IMT has been applied to HF.

2.3. IMT in HF

To date, eight studies using IMT in HF have been published; three were not randomized controlled trials (RCTs). Mancini, Henson, LaManca, Donchez, and Levine (1995) recruited 14 patients with chronic stable HF (Classes II–IV) to participate in a multifaceted training protocol. Eight subjects completed the 3-month supervised program, with 90-minute sessions thrice a week. IMT was performed at 30% of PI_{max} for 20 minutes. PI_{max} significantly increased, and dyspnea during activities improved in most subjects. The comprehensiveness of treatment prevents clear determination of the impact of IMT. Cahalin, Semigran, and Dec (1997) studied 14 patients with chronic HF who were randomly selected from pretransplantation testing. Subjects trained for 5–15 minutes thrice a week for 8 weeks at 20% PI_{max}. Significant improvements in PI_{max}, PE_{max}, and dyspnea were noted on Weeks 2 and 6. Padula and Yeaw (2001) completed two home-based pilot studies of IMT in frail older adults with stable chronic HF. Results supported the ability of this sample to master the technique and to use it safely. These studies are limited by lack of a control group.

The remaining five studies were RCTs, all of which used sham training at 0–15% PI_{max} for control groups and varying pressure loads for treatment groups. All subjects had chronic stable Class II and Class III HF. Johnson, Cowley, and Kinnear (1998) randomized 18 patients into a treatment group or a sham training group. Subjects received daily 30-minute IMT training, with IMT subjects training at 30% PI_{max} versus 15% for control subjects. Sixteen subjects completed the training. PI_{max} increased significantly in the training group as compared to the control group. Exercise tolerance and QOL scores measured by a researcher-developed instrument did not change significantly. Weiner, Waizman, Magadle, Berar-Yanan, and Pelled (1999) randomized 20 subjects into a study group and a sham group. The treatment group received IMT training that increased in 3 months to 60% of PI_{max}. Control subjects trained at 15% of PI_{max} throughout; both trained six times a week for half-hour sessions. Four control subjects dropped out. The IMT group showed a significant increase in PI_{max}, PE_{max}, dyspnea (measured by the Dyspnea Index), and spirometry scores, which were unchanged in the control group. Martinez et al. (2001)

trained 20 subjects at 10% ($n = 9$) or 30% ($n = 11$) PI_{max} for twice-daily 15-minute sessions, 6 days a week for 6 weeks. Both groups showed improved Dyspnea Index scores, maximal oxygen uptake, and PI_{max}, but 6-Minute Walk scores increased in the treatment group only. Laoutaris et al. (2004) used a prospective sex-matched and age-matched controlled study; 35 subjects were recruited and supervised using IMT with computer interface. Twenty subjects trained to respiratory fatigue at 60% of PI_{max}, whereas 17 controls trained at 15%, both thrice a week for 10 weeks. Two control subjects withdrew. The training group showed significantly increased PI_{max}, perceived dyspnea (Borg scale), QOL (Minnesota Living with Heart Failure measure; Recto, Kubo & Cohn, 1986), and walking. The control group also significantly increased PI_{max}. Dall'Ago, Chiappa, Guths, Stein, and Ribeiro (2006) randomized 44 subjects into a 12-week home-based IMT program. Treatment subjects ($n = 16$) trained at 30% PI_{max}, whereas control subjects ($n = 16$) trained daily with no pressure load. Six subjects withdrew from each group. With IMT, PI_{max} increased by 115%; oxygen uptake, PE_{max}, 6-Minute Walk, and Minnesota Living with Heart Failure improved significantly.

In summary, although all five studies used the same target population, they employed widely varying training protocols in terms of PI_{max}, frequency, and duration. All five used sham or placebo training; dropout in the sham training group tended to be higher as subjects became aware of the sham. Varying outcomes were measured with often differing instruments, making generalizations difficult. Although sample sizes were small, statistically significant increases in PI_{max} were detected in all five, although effect sizes were not reported. Training even at suboptimal loads may improve IM strength, although higher levels may achieve more measurable results. It can be concluded that IMT is effective in increasing IM strength in HF. Further research is needed to clearly specify dosing and to determine the impact of IMT on dyspnea and QOL. All of the studies were atheoretical; one RCT (Dall'Ago et al., 2006) was home-based and was conducted by a physical therapist. This research expands and extends previous research using a nurse-coached IMT intervention in the home and based on Self-Efficacy Theory.

3. Framework

Bandura's (1986) Self-Efficacy Theory provided the framework that directed nursing interventions. Self-efficacy refers to people's belief in their capabilities to mobilize the motivation, cognitive resources, and courses of action needed to meet given situational demands. There are four empirically verified ways to enhance self-efficacy: performance accomplishment, vicarious experiences, verbal persuasion, and enactive attainment. These strategies were incorporated and documented during home visits and telephone calls for both groups.

20   *C.A. Padula et al. / Applied Nursing Research 22 (2009) 18–25*

4. Method

4.1. Overall goal and specific aims

The overall goal was to determine the effect of nurse-coached IMT on people with chronic stable HF. The primary aim was to determine the effect of 3 months of nurse-coached IMT with respect to IM strength and perceived dyspnea. The secondary aims were to determine the effect of IMT with respect to self-efficacy for breathing and physical/functional and psychosocial dimensions of HRQOL.

4.2. Research question

The research question is as follows: "Is a home-based IMT intervention more effective in improving IM strength, dyspnea, self-efficacy for breathing, and HRQOL outcomes than an educational comparison group?"

4.3. Research design

This research is a two-group quasiexperimental design with random assignment to groups. Subjects were randomized by a coin toss into either an experimental group (IMT) ($n = 15$) or a control group ($n = 17$), which received a standard educational protocol. Data on PI_{max} (IMT group), Borg scores, blood pressure (BP), heart rate (HR), respiratory rate (RR) and pattern, lung sounds, edema, and weight were collected at six time points: baseline, Week 1, Week 3, Week 6, Week 9, and Week 12; data on the Medical Outcome Study (MOS) 36-item Short Form Health Survey (SF-36), Chronic Respiratory Disease Questionnaire (CRDQ), COPD Self-Efficacy Scale (CSES), and PI_{max} (PE group) were collected at baseline and on Weeks 6 and 12. These data points were based on literature, previous research, clinical knowledge, and principles derived from the Self-Efficacy Theory. The possibility of a testing effect was recognized but minimized by the spacing of testing intervals. Random assignment protected against selection bias. Other inherent threats to internal validity were minimized by: (1) mortality: periodic home visits with telephone calls; (2) maturation/fatigue: IMT intervals and adjustments were based on subjects' physiological tolerance; and (3) instrumentation: research assistants (RAs) were instructed to follow standard protocol in an orderly sequence. The same RA collected data on each subject. To ensure equivalence, the same numbers of home visits, telephone calls, and contact hours were observed. The threat of history can be assumed because, midway through the study, Health Insurance Portability and Accountability Act (HIPPA) guidelines were implemented, which hindered data collection in some areas, particularly in physicians' offices.

The independent variable was the 12-week home IMT intervention. The control group received a patient education (PE) instructional program. The concepts of treatment integrity and treatment fidelity were observed. The aim was to treat the members of the two groups in the same way. Integrity checks were carried out regularly, with frequent monitoring and feedback from the RAs

who were also supervised on the first home visit. The feedback consisted of not only the interventions but also the type of self-efficacy enhancements used. There were uniform orientation and careful training with attention to following the specified protocol, as well as supervision throughout the intervention. Each RA implemented data collection in an ordered sequence to maintain procedural consistency. All data collectors had their own Threshold Device and were required to practice the technique, thereby familiarizing themselves with various sensations. This study was reviewed and approved by three institutional review boards. Recruiting physicians signed the Federal Wide Assurance forms, and RAs completed human subjects certifications.

4.3.1. IMT intervention and compliance

The Threshold Device (Healthscan) was used for resistive IMT breathing training. Its has been widely used successfully in COPD research and, to a lesser degree, with other diagnoses. Training consisted of demonstration by the RAs, with return demonstration at baseline followed by a week of device use. Subjects kept a log noting duration and frequency. RAs noted the intensity on the log and recorded duration and frequency on data collection flow sheets. PI_{max} scores were obtained using a reliability-tested inspiratory force meter, and the mean of scores from five trials was recorded. Then, 30% of that PI_{max} value was calculated and used to calibrate the training load. The Threshold Device was adjusted to 30% of PI_{max} on each home visit. This progression allowed individuals to adapt without muscle soreness but to exercise IMs. Subjects in the experimental group trained 7 days/week, with the exception of one subject who trained 6 days/week. The duration of training varied from 10 to 20 minutes/day, with two subjects who trained twice a day for 10–15 minutes each time. A monitoring instrument was used to validate compliance and to confirm notations on the client's log sheet. The instrument is a box with an internal timer, with tubing attached to one end and the other end attached to a port that hooked onto the mouthpiece. The instrument and protocol were successfully implemented and tested for reliability and validity by and procured through Larson (consultant). The timer monitors the overall number of trials and the time over the period between visits.

4.3.2. Patient education

The control group received a booklet designed by the coinvestigators and a graduate student (Lisa Sullivan, RN, MS) and covered information such as: basic anatomy and physiology of the heart, diet, medication regimen, sleep, rest, and activity patterns, and what and when to report to the doctor. It was designed to observe the principles of teaching adults, incorporated self-efficacy principles, and was at the seventh-grade level according to the Simple Measure of Gobbledygook (SMOG) readability index.

C.A. Padula et al. / Applied Nursing Research 22 (2009) 18–25   21

4.4. Integration of the Self-Efficacy Theory

Bandura's Self-Efficacy Theory guided the interventions for both the experimental group (IMT) and the control group (PE). Vicarious experiences for the IMT group were accomplished by observing the demonstration of the task of using the Threshold Device, thus "modeling" the instruction and demonstration provided by the RA. Performance accomplishment was achieved by "mastering" the technique of inspiring into the device with a nose clip in place. On each subsequent visit, proficiency was increased so that subjects became comfortable. During instruction, verbal persuasion through encouragement, clarification, and reinterpretation occurred with reinforcement upon subsequent visits. Enactive attainment was realized by reexamining prior goals and setting new ones at every visit and by increasing IMT load based on PI_{max} scores, thus providing tangible evidence of progress.

For the control group, performance accomplishment was achieved by "mastering" educational content. At the beginning of each home visit, previous content was reviewed and reinforced (reinterpretation). During the home visit, each subject and the RA reviewed prior goals and identified new ones as needed (enactive attainment). Vicarious experience was the least used strategy, whereas verbal persuasion was the most frequent strategy used in this group. During the 12 weeks, positive verbal persuasion was used for both groups during telephone calls to provide validation, feedback, praise, and reassurance. Both groups were encouraged to maintain a diary (performance accomplishment); the IMT group also kept a log of the duration and frequency of device use. The use of these strategies during home visits and telephone follow-up maintained motivation and fostered compliance.

4.5. Recruitment

Recruitment sites included physicians' offices, home care agencies, provider referral, and newspaper advertisement. Inclusion criteria included the following: (1) adult; (2) community dwelling; (3) stable Class II or III HF with an ejection fraction of < 45%; (4) without coexisting pulmonary disease; and (5) without cognitive impairment as measured by the Mini Mental State Exam. After determining eligibility criteria and obtaining informed consent, potential subjects were randomized into the two groups. It was *estimated* that for every subject who met eligibility criteria, four were eliminated because of COPD comorbidity. In addition, one in every four subjects was excluded because of higher ejection fraction and other health reasons. It was projected, based on similar studies using home intervention in a 12-week period, that a 20% attrition rate would occur. However, subjects in this study, for the most part, were compliant with each of the regimens. One subject withdrew from the IMT group on Week 6 because of time constraints, explaining that he did not like to be "tied down" to a set amount of time for a specific activity. He did request

to be included in the PE program—a request we honored. Another subject withdrew on the eighth week because of death in the family. A third subject withdrew on the ninth week because of busy schedule. All other subjects were compliant throughout the data collection period. As Fig. 1 depicts, 48% of the sampling frame was ineligible because of COPD comorbidity, and 40% was ineligible because of ejection fraction and other factors. Therefore, 13.8% of the subjects who were screened were eligible. Strict eligibility criteria were upheld to maintain the quality of the data.

4.6. Measures

4.6.1. Dependent variables and measures

IMS was measured by obtaining PI_{max} scores according to the universally accepted Black and Hyatt (1969) techniques. PI_{max} is the maximal vacuum pressure generated at the mouth against an occluded airway that is sustained for one full second. The validity of PI_{max} as a measure of IMS is supported by strong correlations between PI_{max} and maximal transdiaphragmatic pressure at $r + .93$ (Braun, Arora & Rochester, 1982). The PI_{max} has high test–retest reliability $[r - .97 \ (df + 89)]$ if sufficient practice is provided to overcome learning effects (Larson et al., 2002). The test–retest reliability of the two inspiratory force meters (using $n = 12$) was established by the investigators at $r = .98$, using a minimum of five trials to obtain the average score for PI_{max}.

Dyspnea was measured by the Borg (1982) scale, which incorporates the use of category methods with ratio properties. The Borg scale provides ratings of perceived exertion on a 0–10 scale, with 0 = *nothing at all* and 10 = *very, very strong*. The rationale for using the Borg scale was based on the belief that it is important to understand subjective symptoms and their relationship to objective parameters; it has high reliability correlations. *Dyspnea intensity and distress* were operationalized using the dyspnea scale of the CRDQ (Guyatt, Berman, Townsend, Pugsley, & Chambers, 1987). The CRDQ elicits subjects' shortness of breath (SOB) due to activities. Subjects are

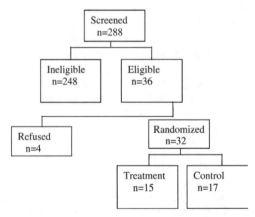

Fig. 1. Recruitment flow chart.

22   *C.A. Padula et al. / Applied Nursing Research 22 (2009) 18–25*

Table 1
Demographic and clinical characteristics of the study sample, by group at baseline

Variable	IMT group (n = 15)	Control group (n = 17)
Gender (male:female)	5:10	7:10
Marital status		
Married	9	8
Divorced	6	6
Widowed		3
Age in years [M (range)]	76 (51–89)	73 (32–95)
NYHA classification		
II	5	9
III	7	6
Mean MOS SF-36 score	29.15	29.11
Mean self-efficacy score	3.11	3.64
Mean CRDQ dyspnea score	3.4	3.6
Mean diastolic BP (mmHg)	70	67
Mean systolic BP (mmHg)	129	131
Mean HR	70	68
Mean RR	23	20
Mean weight (lb)	160	196
Mean PI_{max} (cmH_2O)	48.72	52.25

asked to identify subjectively perceived specific activities that caused SOB within the last 2 weeks, after which they rank ordered the activities important to them. In addition, there is a checklist consisting of an array of usual activities caused by SOB. The process continues until the subjects' degree of dyspnea is noted based on the perceived five most important activities. Subjects are then asked to rate the degree of SOB experienced during the last 2 weeks while they were performing those activities; scores range from 1 = *extremely SOB* to 7 = *not at all SOB*. Test–retest reliability and concurrent reliability have been established. Use was based on the premise that it includes a valid symptom-specific measure of dyspnea that would detect IMT effect and differences in small samples with excellent reproducibility in 12 weeks (Guyatt et al., 1987).

Self-efficacy related to breathing was measured by the CSES, a 34-item measure with good test–retest reliability (r + 0.77) and excellent internal consistency (Cronbach's α = .95) (Wigal, Creer, & Kostes, 1991). Because this scale was used primarily with patients with COPD, we submitted it to a panel of experts to confirm its content validity for use in an HF sample. Ten advanced practice nurses experienced in HF management responded to the questionnaire. Findings were supportive of using the CSES, with modification of the content "when I *am*" to "when I *feel*" in six items. The scale was then piloted using a representative sample of people with HF.

Physical/functional and psychosocial dimensions of HRQOL were measured by the MOS SF-36 (Ware & Sherbourne, 1992). The SF-36 is a multi-item scale consisting of eight health concepts, including physical and mental health functioning. Scores range from 0 to 100; the lower is the score, the greater is the impairment. Both physical and mental components show convergent and discriminant validity (McHorney, Ware, & Raczek, 1993).

Subjects were encouraged to maintain a *diary* on which they could record progress made or issues to be discussed during subsequent phone or home visit contacts.

General demographic data and New York Heart Association (NYHA) classification, a widely used system to classify limitations in ability to perform physical activity, were obtained at baseline.

Clinical assessments during home visits included weight, HR, BP, RR and respiratory pattern, edema, lung sounds, and review of self-reported symptoms. A log was used to collect and document data at baseline, Week 1, Week 3, Week 6, Week 9, and Week 12.

5. Results

5.1. Sample

The demographic characteristics of the two groups are illustrated in Table 1. The mean age was 74.7 years, ranging from 32 to 95 years for both groups. The gender (47% male) and ethnicity (85% White, 9% Hispanic, 3% Black, and 3% Native American) of the sample corresponded closely to those of the state population (48% male, 87% White, and 13% non-White), with the minority population slightly overrepresented in the study. The NYHA classification among the total sample was 51.8% Class II and 48.3% Class III. Baseline scores, including MOS SF-36 (HRQOL), self-efficacy, CRDQ (dyspnea), diastolic and systolic BP, and HR, were comparable in the two groups; there were no statistically significant differences. Baseline PI_{max} scores were lower in the IMT group (42.24 cm) than in the control group (52.25 cm), as were ejection fractions (30.47 {IMT}; 33.24 {PE}). Baseline RR was higher in the IMT group (23) than in the PE group (20), as was weight (160 vs. 196 lb).

5.2. IM strength

PI_{max} in the IMT group increased from 48.72 ± 25.69 at baseline to 78.5 ± 37.08 on Week 12; in the control group,

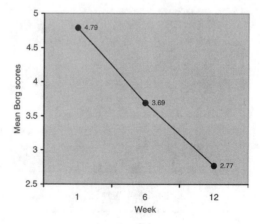

Fig. 2. Mean Borg dyspnea scores: IMT group.

C.A. Padula et al. / Applied Nursing Research 22 (2009) 18–25 23

the PI$_{max}$ remained unchanged (52.25 $\pm$ 27.32; 52.61 $\pm$ 28.25). Repeated measures revealed a significant difference in PI$_{max}$ repeated measures, $F(3,29) = 8.7$, $p < .0001$. To determine where significant differences lie, Tukey (Honestly Significant Differences [HSD]) postanalytic test was performed; scores on Week 1 were significantly different from those on Weeks 9 and 12. Effect size using Cohen's d was .48, a medium effect.

5.3. Dyspnea

Borg scores ($0 = no\ SOB$; $10 = maximal\ SOB$) from baseline to Week 12 were significantly different as evaluated by repeated-measures analysis of variance (ANOVA), Wilk's $\lambda = 0.626$, $F(2,30)=17.36$, $p < .0001$. Post hoc analysis revealed that scores at Time 1 (Week 1) were significantly higher than those at Time 3 (Week 12) (Fig. 2). Dyspnea was also measured using the CDRQ ($1 = extremely\ SOB$; $7 = no\ SOB$). Fig. 3 depicts the results. CRDQ scores increased from baseline in the IMT group. Significant differences were detected in CRDQ scores, as evaluated by repeated-measures ANOVA, Wilk's $\lambda = 0.66$, $F(2,19) = 4.9$, $p = .019$. The five subjectively perceived activities causing SOB were: walking upstairs ($n = 23$), walking uphill ($n = 19$), carrying groceries ($n = 18$), going for a walk ($n = 17$), and hurrying ($n = 17$) (Table 2). Subjects listed from 0 to 20 activities leading to SOB, with a mean of 8. Eleven individuals mentioned that they used pacing/accommodating strategies to decrease their SOB. Rank sum test was used to compare participants' rankings of SOB on the three activities identified as most important to them. Rankings were compared by group for Time 1 (baseline), Time 2 (6 weeks), and Time 3 (12 weeks). Differences between the study group (IMT) and the control group (PE) on rankings for two of the three most important activities at Times 2 and 3 were statistically significant ($p = .027$, Activity 1, Time 2; $p = .046$, Activity 1, Time 3; $p = .011$, Activity 2, Time 2; $p < .001$, Activity 2, Time 3). Participants in the IMT group demonstrated significantly less SOB during two of the three self-identified most

Table 2
Frequency of subjectively perceived activities causing SOB (CRDQ)

Activity	n
Walking upstairs	23
Walking uphill	19
Carrying	18
Going for a walk	17
Hurrying	17
Bending	16
Walking with others on level ground	14
Making bed	12
Shopping	12
Vacuuming	11
Housework	10
Lying flat	8
Mopping floor	7
Walking around own home	7
While trying to sleep	7
Being angry or upset	6
Running	6
Talking	6
Moving furniture	5
Playing with children or grandchildren	5
Dressing	4
Eating	3
Playing sports	3
Reaching over the head	2
Preparing meals	1

Notes. Other activities/conditions perceived by individuals to cause SOB included the following: bicycling (1), humidity (1), lifting (1), singing (1), cutting grass (1), and snow shoveling (1).

important activities at 6 and 12 weeks as compared to subjects in the PE group.

5.4. Physical/functional and psychosocial HRQOL; self-efficacy

Scores from the MOS SF-26 and the SES were not significantly different.

5.5. Respiratory rate

RR was significantly different between groups, as measured by mixed between/within ANOVA, $F(1,20) = 6.2$, $p. = .02$; within-subject means on the repeated measure (time) were not significant.

5.6. Other findings

A serendipitous finding was noted at midpoint. Several subjects in both groups mentioned that they had intended to go to or call their doctor's office but refrained from doing so because a home visit or telephone call was pending. These occurrences were thereafter noted among four subjects.

6. Discussion

The critical dependent variables of IMS and dyspnea, as operationalized by three measures, provide support that IMT as a home intervention with nurse coaching can be a therapeutic intervention in clients with Class II and III HF.

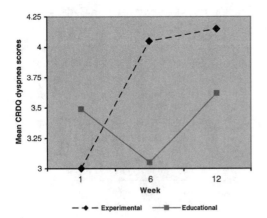

Fig. 3. Mean CRDQ dyspnea scores by week: IMT and educational groups.

The results of improvement in IM strength and endurance as measured by PI_{max} scores are consistent with those of previous researchers. In this study, increases of 64.39% on Week 3, 55% on Week 6, 43.55% on Week 9, and 11.24% on Week 12 were noted. From Weeks 1 to 12, PI_{max} scores increased by 75% in the experimental group. This study had similar results in decreasing Borg dyspnea scores. The dramatic increase in PI_{max} at the beginning of the intervention could be due to a training effect as noted by Cahalin et al. (1997). The gradual decrease over time in the percentage of change could be attributed to the training load with a resistance of 30% of PI_{max}. Positive results from the CDRQ and the Borg scale, both of which measured dyspnea, are encouraging; perhaps more important was the finding that IMT subjects reported significantly less SOB on Weeks 6 and 12 on two of three self-identified most important activities. CDRQ responses clearly demonstrate the beneficial effect of IMT, where improvement was noted in SOB scores on Weeks 6 and 12.

The primary aims of this study were achieved although the secondary aims were not. It could be that the use of a generic tool (SF-36) to measure QOL was not sufficiently sensitive to detect changes in subjects' conditions; Laoutaris et al. (2004) and Dall'Ago et al. (2006) demonstrated improvements in QOL as measured by the Minnesota Living with Heart Failure, an HF-specific measure. There is limited research evaluating QOL as a separate variable as distinguished from dyspnea, and it is difficult to capture QOL in people with dyspnea. Further concept analysis and construct validity study would be beneficial. Although the content validity of the CSES was evaluated and deemed appropriate, the semantics used was problematic. An introductory stem asks how confident individuals are in managing or avoiding breathing difficulty in situations, and many subjects had trouble relating confidence to particular situations/activities.

This study was the first RCT to implement nurse-coached, home-based, theoretically driven IMT intervention. The attrition rate from this study (6.2%; both from the IMT group) fared well compared with previous researchers studying IMT among people with HF: Mancini et al. (1995), 42.8%; Cahalin et al. (1997), 0%; Johnson et al. (1998), 11.1%; Weiner et al. (1999), 20%; Laoutaris et al. (2004), 5.7%; Martinez et al. (2001), none reported. Compliance as validated by the monitoring instrument, although an estimate revealed close approximation to reported log frequencies and times. Also supporting compliance is that IMT is relatively easy to learn and has been successfully mastered by people across a wide variety of conditions. Consistent with other research, subjects had no reported difficulty in mastering the technique.

7. Limitations and recommendations

The sample size was relatively small, although in comparison to similar studies, this research generated a respectable sample size ($n = 31$): Cahalin et al. (1997), $n =$ 14; Mancini et al. (1995), $n = 14$; Johnson et al. (1998), $n = 27$; Weiner et al. (1999), $n = 20$; Laoutaris et al. (2004), $n = 35$; Martinez et al. (2001), $n = 20$. Although patient logs and diaries were useful, they were not universally used, perhaps because of the frequent telephone calls and home visits. Recommendations for future research include the following: including subjects with COPD and HF comorbidity as a comparison group because that combination is prominent in the population; tracking the number of doctors' visits and telephone calls preventing emergency room and physician office visits; using a different tool to measure self-efficacy; and evaluating the effects of varying intensity loads. This study has provided evidence that home-based IMT can be effective in improving dyspnea and IM strength. However, improvement in QOL and self-efficacy (for breathing) remains questionable. Thus, the primary aims were achieved but not the secondary aims; further study is needed.

8. Clinical application

The extensive IMT research that has accumulated across clinical conditions has established IMT as a safe and effective intervention to improve IMS; this research extended IMT to a theoretically driven, nurse-coached, home-based intervention. Clinical application of IMT in HF has potential as an adjuvant therapy, along with medication regimens and rehabilitation. Currently, IMT is not widely seen in clinical nursing practice; because the Threshold Device is a medical device, use is restricted to trained health care professionals. Medicare has previously funded the Threshold Device for use in COPD but not at present. However, a variety of IM training devices are now readily available to consumers via the Internet and are being advocated for a variety of purposes. The cost is of an IMT training device, which can be used in the long term with regular cleaning, is about US$25.

Numerous clinical implications can be derived from this study. A strength was that nurses regularly performed in-depth physical assessment, including vital signs, lung sounds, and weight monitoring, in addition to designated outcome measures. This hands-on approach not only provided invaluable information but also helped to establish credibility and trust with subjects. Although not part of the research protocol, the research nurse frequently made telephone contact with physicians to report, clarify, or report and clarify health status. Physicians identified this as a strength, and some believed that these exchanges prevented hospitalization. The value of telephone follow-up was clearly supported in data collection, providing support and maintaining motivation in subjects. Telephone monitoring, particularly when performed consistently by a nurse familiar with the individual's history, is an invaluable resource for both the nurse and the patient.

Application of the constructs derived from the Self-Efficacy Theory was extremely effective; strategies can be

C.A. Padula et al. / Applied Nursing Research 22 (2009) 18–25 25

applied in a wide variety of clinical settings. The use of mutual goal setting was identified as particularly beneficial and was a key component of the intervention. Nurses worked actively with subjects to formulate client-centered, realistic, and achievable goals. Goals provided a benchmark to strive toward, as well as positive reinforcement for progress achieved, discussed at each contact, and updated and modified as indicated. Symptom interpretation was carefully integrated throughout the intervention and can be applied to most clinical situations. Verbal persuasion, gently coaxing individuals while providing accurate information and support in a trusting environment, can be very helpful. Using vicarious experiences, nurses can assist people to adapt to disease states by learning from others' experiences. It is important to note that the researchers were not restrained by time during home visits, which is a unique circumstance not familiar to practicing nurses today. However, it is believed that many of these strategies can be effectively integrated within the demands of delivering quality nursing care.

Acknowledgment

This research was supported by an AREA (Academic Research Enhancement Award) grant from the National Institute of Nursing Research (R15NR08077-01). The authors acknowledge Janet Larson, PhD, FAAN, who served as a consultant throughout this project. The authors also acknowledge graduate assistant support provided by the College of Nursing, University of Rhode Island, specifically the work of Kathy Gremel, RN, MS, Lisa Sullivan, RN, MS, and Jeiny Zapata, RN, MS.

References

American Heart Association. (2000). AHA scientific statement. Team management of patients with heart failure. *Circulation, 102*, 2443–2456.

Bandura, A. (1986). *Social foundations of thought and action: A social cognitive theory.* Englewood Cliffs, NJ: Prentice-Hall.

Black, L. F., & Hyatt, P. E. (1969). Maximal respiratory pressures: Normal values and relationship to age and sex. *American Review Respiratory Disease, 99*, 696–702.

Borg, G. (1982). Psychophysical bases of perceived exertion. *Medicine and Science in Sports and Exercise, 14*(5), 377–381.

Braun, N., Arora, N., & Rochester, D. (1982). Force–length relationship of the normal human diaphragm. *Journal of Applied Physiology, 53*(2), 405–412.

Cahalin, L., Semigran, M., & Dec, G. (1997). Inspiratory muscle training in patients with chronic heart failure awaiting cardiac transplantation. *Physical Therapy, 77*(8), 830–838.

Caroci, A., & Lareau, S. (2004). Descriptors of dyspnea by patients with chronic obstructive pulmonary disease versus congestive heart failure. *Heart & Lung, 33*(2), 102–110.

Clark, A., Poole-Wilson, P., & Coats, A. (1996). Exercise limitation in chronic heart failure: Central role of the periphery. *Journal of the American College of Cardiology, 28*, 1092–1102.

Dall'Ago, P., Chiappa, G., Guths, H., Stein, R., & Ribeiro, J. (2006). Inspiratory muscle raining in patients with heart failure and inspiratory muscle weakness. *Journal of the American College of Cardiology, 47*(4), 757–763.

Gibbs, J., Keegan, J., Wright, C., Fox, K., & Poole-Wilson, P. (1990). Pulmonary artery pressure changes during exercise and daily activities in chronic heart failure. *Journal of the American College of Cardiology, 15*, 52–61.

Guyatt, G., Berman, L., Townsend, M., Pugsley, S., & Chambers, L. (1987). A measure of quality of life for clinical trials in chronic lung disease. *Thorax, 42*, 773–778.

Johnson, P., Cowley, A., & Kinnear, W. (1998). A randomized controlled trial of inspiratory muscle training in stable chronic heart failure. *European Heart Journal, 19*, 1249–1253.

Larson, J., Covey, M., & Corbridge, S. (2002). Inspiratory muscle strength in chronic obstructive pulmonary disease. *AACN Clinical Issues, 13*(2), 320–332.

Larson, J., & Kim, K. (1987). Ineffective breathing pattern related to respiratory muscle fatigue. *Nursing Clinics of North America, 22*, 207–223.

Laoutaris, I., Dritsas, A., Brown, M., Manginas, A., Alivizatos, P., & Cokkinos, D. (2004). Inspiratory muscle training using an incremental endurance test alleviates dyspnea and improves functional status in patients with chronic heart failure. *Eur J Cardiovasc Prev Rehabil, 11*(6), 489–496.

Mancini, D., Henson, D., LaManca, J., Donchez, L., & Levine, S. (1995). Benefit of selective respiratory muscle training on exercise capacity in patients with chronic congestive heart failure. *Circulation, 91*, 320–329.

Martinez, A., Lisboa, C., Jalil, J., Munoz, V., Diaz, O., Casanegra, P., et al. (2001). Selective training of respiratory muscles in patients with heart failure. *Revista Medica de Chile, 129*(2), 133–139.

McConnell, T., Mandak, J., Sykes, J., Fesniak, H., & Dasgupta, H. (2003). Exercise training for heart failure patients improves respiratory muscle endurance, exercise tolerance, breathlessness, and quality of life. *Journal of Cardiopulmonary Rehabilitation, 23*(1), 10–16.

McHorney, C., Ware, J., & Raczek, A. B. (1993). The MOS 36-item Short Form Health Survey (SF-36): II. Psychometric and clinical tests of validity in measuring physical and mental constructs. *Medical Care, 31*(3), 247–263.

Padula, C., & Yeaw, E. (2001). Inspiratory muscle training: An exploration of a home-based intervention. *Journal of Applied Research, 1*(2), 85–94.

Rector, T., Kubo, S., & Cohn, J. (1986). Patients' self assessment of their congestive heart failure: Part 2. Content, reliability, and validity of a new measure, the Minnesota Living with Heart Failure questionnaire. *Heart Failure, 3*, 198–209.

Rogers, F. (2001). The muscle hypothesis: A model for chronic heart failure appropriate for osteopathic medicine. *Journal of the American Osteopathic Association, 101*(10), 576–583.

Vibarel, N., Hayot, M., Ledermann, B., Pellenc, P., Ramonatxo, M., & Prefaut, C. (2002). Effect of aerobic exercise training on inspiratory muscle performance and dyspnoea in patients with chronic heart failure. *European Journal of Heart Failure, 4*, 745–751.

Ware, J., & Sherbourne, C. (1992). The MOS 36-item Short-Form Health Survey (SF-36). *Medical Care, 30*(6), 473–481.

Weiner, P., Waizman, J., Magadle, R., Berar-Yanay, N., & Pelled, B. (1999). The effect of specific inspiratory muscle training on the sensation of dyspnea and exercise tolerance in patients with congestive heart failure. *Clinical Cardiology, 22*, 727–732.

Wigal, J., Creer, T., & Kotses, H. (1991). The COPD Self-Efficacy Scale. *Chest, 99*, 1193–1196.

Nursing Research • January/February 2010 • Vol 59, No 1, 11–17

Online Fathering

The Experience of First-Time Fatherhood in Combat-Deployed Troops

Kathleen A. Schachman

Editor's Note

Materials documenting the review process for this article are posted at
http://www.nursing-research-editor.com

▶ **Background:** More than 90% of fathers in the United States attend the births of their children. Each year, thousands of fathers are absent during this important life transition because of military deployment in combat regions; however, it is unknown how this population experiences new fatherhood.

▶ **Objective:** The purpose of this study was to explore the lived experience of first-time fatherhood from the unique perspective of military men deployed to combat regions during birth.

▶ **Method:** A phenomenological approach was used. Seventeen men who were stationed in Okinawa, Japan, and had returned recently from a combat deployment participated. Unstructured, in-depth interviews were conducted 2 to 6 months after the births. Interviews were audiotaped, transcribed, and analyzed using Colaizzi's method.

▶ **Results:** *Disruption of the protector and provider role* was a main theme that encompassed four theme clusters: (a) worry—a traumatic and lonely childbirth; (b) lost opportunity; (c) guilt—an absent father; and (d) fear of death and dismemberment—who will be the father? Although their absence interfered with their ability to fulfill the fatherhood role as they perceived it, this was offset by the theme cluster *Communication: The ties that bind*, highlighting the role of online communication with their partner (e.g., e-mail, instant messaging, Facebook™, blogs, and chat rooms) in restoring balance to the protector and provider role.

▶ **Discussion:** Insight is provided into the needs of first-time fathers who are combat-deployed during the births of their babies. Understanding these experiences assists nurses in identifying better ways to prepare and to support men in an involved fatherhood role, despite the limitations of a stressful combat environment and geographic separation. This information can set the stage for a healthy reunion, which may take place at military bases and within communities across the globe, and thus is of benefit to all nurses working with military families.

▶ **Key Words:** childbirth · fatherhood · military · paternal role

O ver the past three decades, men have become a virtually universal presence in the delivery room. Birth attendance by fathers is a culturally prescribed expectation in the United States (Knoester, Petts, & Eggebeen, 2007; Lamb, 2003). The father's presence during childbirth is thought to impact not only maternal outcomes such as the labor process and satisfaction (Essex & Pickett, 2008; Hodnett, Gates, Hofmeyer, & Sakala, 2007) but also family well-being and the development of a favorable father–child relationship (Pleck & Masciadrelli, 2004; Premberg, Hellstrom, & Berg, 2008). Today, over 90% of fathers in the United States attend the birth of their children, and the few fathers who are not present are almost exclusively men who are not in a close relationship with the baby's mother (Reed, 2005). An exception to this, however, is men in the military who are separated geographically from their laboring partners due to combat deployment. Over 100,000 service members are deployed currently in combat regions; more than half of them are married and below the age of 30 years (Department of Defense, Statistical Information Analysis Division, 2009).

Although the preponderance of research concerning fathers' birth attendance has been focused on the effects of their participation on the labor process and on maternal well-being, very little research has explored the father's perspective of this experience. In the handful of studies available, men are described as feeling fearful, excluded, and ill prepared for the birth event (Deave & Johnson, 2008; Johnson, 2002; Rosich-Medina & Shetty, 2007). In a theoretical analysis of men's experiences during labor and birth, Draper (2003) observed: "Labor was a particularly ambiguous time for men. Although invited into the labor room, most felt out of place, powerless, unsure of what to do, and therefore very vulnerable" (p. 70). However, for many men, incorporation into the new role as a father begins with childbirth. The ritual of seeing the birth

Kathleen A. Schachman, PhD, APRN-BC, is Associate Professor, Montana State University, Bozeman.

facilitates the onset of the social transition to fatherhood (Draper, 2003). In a sociocultural analysis of fatherhood, Barclay and Lupton (1999) noted that a sense of responsibility and protectiveness frequently emerged immediately after birth. For many new fathers, the birth evoked strong emotions and a feeling of connection with the newborn (Goodman, 2005), as the father sought to claim his baby by identifying personal or familial features (Jordan, 1990).

Although important insight into the father's perspectives of childbirth has been demonstrated, the perspective of men who are absent during this important event remains unknown. Members of the military are separated from their families frequently, and often these critical life transitions occur during their absence. Furthermore, for many military members, the childbirth event may occur in the context of a combat deployment. Because most of these new fathers anticipate returning to the family and assuming an active parenting role, it is critical to have an understanding of their needs and perspectives. Better understanding of new fatherhood in this population may inform more helpful and supportive approaches to facilitating fathers' participation in the new role, despite the challenges of a stressful combat environment and geographic separation. The purpose of this qualitative study was to explore the lived experience of first-time fatherhood from the unique perspective of military men who are deployed to combat regions during birth.

Methods

Study Design

A descriptive phenomenological design using the methods of Colaizzi (1978) was used to further the understanding of first-time fatherhood in combat-deployed troops. A phenomenological approach is well suited for this study because the focus is on the lived experience from the perspective of the informants and because little is known about this experience.

Setting and Sample

Purposive sampling was used for recruitment of eligible participants. Men stationed in Okinawa, Japan, who were attending a postdeployment briefing and self-identified as first-time fathers were invited to participate. Recruitment continued until saturation was achieved.

Procedures

Approval from the university's institutional review board was granted prior to the study. After obtaining informed consent from each father, an open-ended interview was conducted by the researcher at the father's home. Each man was asked a single question: "What is it like to become a father while deployed overseas to a combat region?" Follow-up questions were used only as required for clarification. All interviews lasted from 40 to 65 minutes and were audiotaped. Following each interview, field notes were recorded to document observations about the father and the environment. Audiotaped interviews and field notes were transcribed verbatim within 72 hours.

Data Analysis

The interviews were analyzed using the phenomenological process of analysis described by Colaizzi (1978); these steps of analysis are presented in Table 1. Each transcribed interview and the field notes were read several times to gain a sense of the whole experience of each man. After a line-by-line analysis, 182 significant phrases and statements were highlighted and extracted. Each significant statement was studied very carefully to determine the meaning, and through an interpretive process, formulated meanings were derived (Table 2). The formulated meanings were arranged into clusters of themes with common meanings, and the theme clusters were integrated into a description of the essential structure of the phenomenon. At each point, the interpretive decision-making process was shared with a peer researcher to verify the accuracy of the formulated meanings and emerging themes. In general, this led to agreement and confirmation; however, if a discrepancy in interpretation existed, both met and reviewed the data until agreement was achieved.

Trustworthiness

The central goal in maintaining rigor in qualitative inquiry is to represent participants' experiences correctly as reported (Streubert & Carpenter, 1999). This goal was achieved in this study through prolonged engagement with the data, verification with participant feedback, using extracts from participants' verbatim accounts, and peer debriefing. Providing evidence of an audit trail and ensuring technical accuracy in recording and transcribing were strategies used to increase the reliability of the procedures and data generated.

TABLE 1. Steps of Data Analysis
1. Read each participant's verbatim transcript to form an overall impression and acquire a sense of the whole.
2. Extract significant statements by focusing on those aspects seen as most relevant to the phenomenon.
3. Formulate meanings from each of the significant statements, in the context of the participant's terms. Repeat Steps 1–3 with each interview.
4. Organize the meanings from the collective interviews into themes; these themes evolve into theme clusters, and eventually into theme categories.
5. Create an exhaustive description of the phenomenon by integrating the participant's feelings and perceptions of each theme category.
6. Formulate the fundamental structure of the phenomenon.
7. Conduct a member check by taking the findings back to the participants to see if the researcher has adequately captured the essence of the phenomenon.

Note. From Colaizzi (1978).

Nursing Research   January/February 2010 Vol 59, No 1

TABLE 2. Examples of Significant Statements and Corresponding Formulated Meanings Leading to the Theme Cluster "Fear of Death and Dismemberment: Who Will Be the Father?"

Significant statements	Formulated meaning
I remember when [fellow Marine] died. I starting thinking, "Holy cow, that could have been me." I didn't sleep all night, thinking about that, worrying. I kept picturing the Chaplain going to our house, telling [my wife] that I was dead. Her and the baby alone.	When his friend was killed, he thought about his own mortality. He worried about how his wife would receive the news and the prospect of her and the baby being alone.
I worried every day. I was afraid I would not make it back. Sure, money-wise they would be okay I have plenty of [military life insurance]. But who would raise him? Make sure he stayed out of trouble? I am his father that is MY job. I need to get home, I need to get home that is all I could think about.	Although his death would leave them financially secure, he worried that others would assume his role as father.
Dying would be bad but worse than that what if you got totally [maimed]? Like I'm supposed to throw a football to my son with no arms? And then someone has to take care of ME for the rest of my life like I'm a baby?	He felt that a serious injury would be worse than death, and that he would be unable to engage in physical activities with his child, and would be dependent on others for his physical care.
One of the biggest things I worried about was getting a serious injury, you know, like a major head injury or losing both your legs. If something like that happens, you are worse off than dead. You have to depend on other people, and have no way to support your family.	He worried about serious injury. He felt that it was better to die than to become seriously maimed. If he was maimed, he would be dependent on others for financial support and physical care.
Being a father is about supporting your family financially, I mean. If something happens, if I get my arms or legs blown off, there is no way I can support my family. In fact, I would be a burden to them.	His role as financial provider was threatened by the prospect of a serious injury. He would be a burden to his family if he experienced a serious physical injury.
If something happens to me, you know, like lose my legs how would I support my family? I couldn't be a Marine anymore with no legs. I worried about that constantly.	His role as financial provider was threatened by the prospect of a serious injury. He worried that he would lose his job and be unable to support his family if he was seriously injured.

The researcher undertook the process of *bracketing*, a common technique used to ensure that rigor is not compromised due to researcher bias. This was accomplished by first identifying any preconceived assumptions and beliefs held about the phenomenon and through journal writing before and during the data collection and analysis stages. In addition, a peer researcher who had no previous contact with the population or the phenomenon of interest served as a mentor.

Results

Sample

The final sample size consisted of 17 men who had returned recently from combat deployment in the Middle East. Duration of the combat deployment ranged from 6 to 10 months, and all men reported the birth of a first child during the deployment. Interviews were conducted within 1 month of their return, at which time the newborns were 2 to 6 months of age. All of the men were married and had a minimum of a high school education. Nearly 60% ($n = 10$) had at least 2 years of college. The mean age was 23 years ($SD = 2.3$; range = 19 to 26 years). Racial and ethnic breakdown was as follows: 10 Caucasians (59%), 4 African Americans (23%), 2 Hispanic (12%), and 1 other (6%).

Theme Clusters

Five theme clusters emerged that were subsumed under two main themes of *disruption of protector and provider role* and *restoration of the protector and provider role*. The essence of the experience of first-time fatherhood in men deployed to combat regions is captured in these two main themes. Pseudonyms are used in the narrative.

Main Theme 1: Disruption of Protector and Provider Role

The overarching feeling expressed by the new fathers was one of not living up to expectations as they defined the role of fatherhood. They felt an obligation to protect and to provide for their wives and children, and their absence interfered with their ability to fulfill this role. The theme clusters subsumed under this main theme include the following: (a) worry—a traumatic and lonely childbirth; (b) lost opportunity; (c) guilt—an absent father; and (d) fear of death and dismemberment—who will be the father?

Worry: A Traumatic and Lonely Childbirth   During the weeks leading up to the anticipated delivery date, the expectant fathers were consumed with worry. The distressing thoughts and emotions were focused most often on the impending birth. The men described very vivid scenarios in which the normal course of childbirth went awry, and events quickly

Nursing Research January/February 2010 Vol 59, No 1

deteriorated into a scene of turmoil, chaos, and bloodshed. Their imagined role was that of restoring order to a chaotic and dangerous situation. However, in their absence, they were uncertain who would perform that role and were concerned about the safety of their wives and unborn children.

> I kept thinking that something would go really bad during delivery. That for some reason she wouldn't be able to make a decision herself, like if she was unconscious or something. Then the doctor is yelling, "Where's the father, where's the father?" and no one is there for her. No one at all.

Although most of the expectant mothers planned to have support during labor (generally other military wives), the men worried about whether these individuals would serve as adequate substitutes to advocate for the wives' needs and to provide support.

> Someone has to speak up for you, make sure that you get the care that you need... that you deserve... and not just ignored because nobody is there who is willing to do that on your behalf.

Worry often was exacerbated by sporadic and unpredictable access to communication. Lapses in communication spurred anxiety, especially as the due date approached.

> Every day I would check my e-mail. She would send little reports each day. Then for two days nothing! I was out of my mind. I imagined the worst, but of course everything was fine. But it was a bad feeling, not knowing what was going on, because you automatically think the worst.

> I guess she tried to call for three days. Finally, Red Cross sent a message. When the [Officer of the Day] told me I had a Red Cross message, I almost threw up I just knew something bad had happened. I never knew anyone who got a Red Cross message, but I think they're always bad news, not good.

Lost Opportunity Missing the childbirth event was considered a lost opportunity; the men regretted that they were unable to participate in this important life transition. In their idealistic imaginings, they had envisioned a far different scenario, one in which they played an active role in supporting labor, welcoming a new child, and beginning family life together. "Ever because we found out she was pregnant, I have been thinking about how it would be in the delivery room—to suddenly become a father. It's kind of a disappointment that it didn't work out."

Another aspect of lost opportunity pertained to conceptualization of the birth event as the unique time to forge a bond with the new baby. The men worried that their absence would interfere with their ability to connect with the babies and for the babies to connect with and to identify them as the fathers. Raymond worried about how this would influence his daughter's acceptance of him, and he feared rejection:

> I wondered how it would be, meeting her for the first time when she was almost four months old. All the

sudden I show up "who is this guy?" I was worried that she would cry, or worse, be scared of me.

Guilt: An Absent Father Guilt was another theme cluster that served to disrupt the protector and to provider role. The conflict between duty to their chosen profession and duty to their pregnant wives formed the basis for these sentiments. As partners to their wives and as fathers to the unborn children, the men felt an obligation to be present during the birth. These guilt feelings were expressed more intensely by men who felt they had chosen their career consciously above family obligations. Although most had no choice in accepting deployment orders, others actively sought opportunities to deploy—primarily because of enhanced promotion potential, increased pay, or a sense of patriotic duty. Although the selection of career over family often was made with the interest of the family at heart, this still elicited remorse.

> It was a really hard decision should I re-up [re-enlist]? If I re-up, I know I'm going back to Iraq. If I get out, I have a pregnant wife, no health insurance, and no job. Obviously, I re-up'ed. Seemed like the right decision at the time, but maybe I should've taken my chances getting out.

The concept of guilt was expressed also in relation to reliance on others. They acknowledged that their absence placed an additional burden on friends and family. Although they were grateful for the material and emotional support of others, they felt indebted. In addition, the support from others seemingly diminished their paternal role in terms of their ability to protect and to provide for their wives and new children. Often, this sentiment was expressed as a failure to live up to expectations. "Other folks were having to pitch in 'cause I wasn't there. If I were there, she wouldn't have to ask everybody else for help. Just doing simple stuff like going to get groceries."

Finally, expressions of guilt were associated with the expectant fathers' preoccupation with the dynamic combat environment. The periodic and the unpredictable exposure to intense danger blunted their awareness of the lives and families that were going on without them, a half a world away. According to Ryan, to ruminate on thoughts of family life distracted from situational awareness of the combat environment and could put themselves and others at great peril.

> My wife and [unborn] kid were completely off the radar. That really bothered me, that I could completely wipe them from my mind. It made me wonder if that was what kind of father I was going to be. I don't want to be like that someone who totally forgets they have a wife and baby.

Fear of Death and Dismemberment Who Will Be the Father? All of the new fathers feared that they would not return home. The specter of death was a continual presence and a very real threat. The sights and sounds of war were commonplace, and all of the participants had known or heard of other troops who had died during the period they were deployed.

> I remember when [fellow Marine] died. I starting thinking, "Holy cow, that could have been me." I didn't sleep all night, thinking about that, worrying. I kept

Nursing Research January/February 2010 Vol 59, No 1

picturing the Chaplain going to our house, telling [my wife] that I was dead. Her and the baby   alone.

The overarching concern related to death was focused on the fear that they would be abandoning their families, who would be left to struggle on alone. Others were fearful that with death, they would be replaced.

I just can't even picture some other guy bringing up my daughter. Seriously, I don't think anyone else could love her like I would. It's just a biological thing   you'd always love your own kid more than someone else's.

Although they all worried about the welfare of their families should they be killed in combat, they also were afraid that they would never have a chance to see or to hold their new children and that their children would never have a chance to know them: "If I died, he wouldn't even know anything about me—I'm just some guy in a picture, no different than looking at some stranger in a magazine."

Fear of dismemberment or disability was also at the forefront of their concerns. To many, returning home disabled was a more heinous possibility than not returning at all. Gruesome tales of life-altering injuries were shared by each of the men, and they used these as a basis for their belief that death was a preferable alternative. The fear associated with disability was focused on three areas: becoming a burden to their families, being incapable of providing a means to financially support their families, and a perceived inability to raise a child if they were less than whole.

Dying would be bad   but what if you got totally [maimed]? Like I'm supposed to throw a football to my son with no arms? And then someone has to take care of ME for the rest of my life like I'm a baby?

Main Theme 2: Restoration of the Protector and Provider Role

The men's belief that their role as protectors and providers was threatened was balanced by a final theme cluster pertaining to communication.

Communication: The Ties that Bind The men related experiences to highlight the role of communication with their partners in facilitating assumption of the paternal role. Before delivery, frequent communication reassured the men that events were progressing normally, and allayed anxiety, particularly as the delivery dates approached. Fears were put at ease by periodic updates of the expectant mother's condition. Generally, the expectant fathers learned of the birth via e-mail or telephone. Reactions ranged from relief, to joy, and to disbelief.

We were three days without e-mail, so I was nuts the whole time. Sure enough, as soon as I logged on I saw about 10 e-mails. "I'm in labor" or "My water broke," then finally an e-mail from her mom telling me [my son] was born and everyone was just fine. Then, I was kind of glad we were offline for those three days, because if I would've known she was in labor, then I think it would've made it worse. So it was kind of a nice surprise to log on and find out he already arrived! It didn't really sink in until I saw him. [My wife] sent some

e-mail pictures right after delivery. Then it was, like, "Wham! I'm a dad!"

I knew she was in labor. I asked the [Officer of the Day] to come get me as soon as she called. I tried to go to sleep to make the time go by faster, but I couldn't doze off. I was really glad when the [Officer of the Day] finally came to get me. It was so good to hear her voice. I could hear the baby in the background.

After delivery, communication played an essential role in acquainting fathers with their babies, not only detailing mundane day-to-day happenings but also involving them in important child care decisions.

Sometimes something wouldn't be going right, and she'd ask me [via e-mail] what should she do. Like right at the beginning, she was having trouble [breast] feeding the baby, and she says, "Maybe I should just switch to bottle   what do you think?" So, it made me feel like even though I wasn't there that I had some say in the decision, you know, like I was included.

Although e-mail was the most commonly used communication strategy, couples sought increasingly creative means to stay in touch. Antonio watched a video of his son's first bath on YouTube. Spontaneous, real-time communication often occurred through instant messaging. This synchronous, text-based communication allowed both parties to exchange messages because they were able to send messages back and forth privately if both were online simultaneously. Frequently, the time difference made this difficult, so couples would plan a time to be online together so that communication could occur.

Sometimes she would be up in the middle of the night, like if the baby was awake or something. Then suddenly "bing" she pops up on my buddy list [indicating she is online]. So I chime on, find out how she's doing, how did her day go. See what [my daughter] is doing. It was nice to know what was going on over there   it made me feel a little less like an outsider.

Couples also used free-access social networking Web sites such as FacebookTM™ and MySpace™ to stay connected. Jeremy described how his wife expanded her personal profile to include photos and amusing anecdotes about his daughter. She also included links to several Web sites that were geared toward new fathers, with the intent to better prepare him to assume father-related duties upon his return.

I think if I was just going home "cold"   you know, if I didn't get to talk to her all the time, I would've been really nervous … not knowing what to expect. But talking to her online and on the phone really helped both of us. You know, we kind of figured stuff out on our own together, just like we would've if I had been home. Plus, I got to know my son a little bit, even if it was just pictures. It wasn't so bad.

Although Jeremy expressed concern that when he returned home that he would be "a real novice," the links to fathering and baby-care Web sites spurred his confidence. Kenneth also felt that the extensive communication made him feel prepared for his return home for his eventual first introduction to his son.

Discussion

In the eyes of these men, separation from their spouses during childbirth disrupted what they considered to be their primary role as husbands and fathers—that of protector and provider. The interaction of worry, loss, guilt, and fear all disrupted the fulfillment of this role. Psychological distress in expectant and new fathers is not a new concept. Johnson (2002) found that fear is a strong tenet of men's experience of childbirth, with 80% of men reporting fears associated with witnessing the partner's pain, fetal birth injuries, helplessness, and powerlessness. For the men in this study, worry was focused on their inability to control events and to ensure the safety of their wives and babies during childbirth. An interesting finding was that several of the men imagined very vivid and gory near-death childbirth scenarios—whether this can be attributed to their lack of knowledge about the realities of childbirth (none had ever witnessed a birth) or their continuous exposure to a brutal combat environment is worthy of further exploration.

Participants also lacked confidence in healthcare providers and neighbors to serve as adequate substitutes in their absence and believed that they alone could see to the welfare of their loved ones. However, a Cochrane review of 16 randomized trials involving over 13,000 women in 11 countries demonstrated that continuous labor support by other women led to positive birth and psychosocial outcomes for the laboring woman (Hodnett et al., 2007). In response to the unique needs of military wives during childbirth, a number of doula organizations have evolved to serve this population. Anecdotal evidence about doula services for military wives suggests that they confer the same maternal benefits, yet how utilization of doula care impacts a deployed father has not been examined.

The men universally expressed a sense of loss and guilt. Missing the birth of a first child was an important event, and they felt that their physical absence precluded an important opportunity to bond with their newborn. Draper (2003) described labor as a period during which "the man literally became a father, his closeness to a biological transition being intensified within a broader social transition" (p. 70). Yet many new fathers describe the period after the birth as a "blur of exhilaration and exhaustion" and "being in a minor state of shock... totally spaced out" (Draper, 2003, p. 71). In a sociocultural analysis of new fatherhood, Barclay and Lupton (1999) observed that attachment to the newborn is a more gradual process, and that new fathers were often surprised that bonding was not achieved immediately. The guilt expressed by the men included the preconceived notion that they would be present to share in this monumental life-changing event. Societal pressure for men to participate in childbirth may

> *In the eyes of these men, separation from their spouses during childbirth disrupted what they considered to be their primary role as husbands and as fathers.*

have been a contributing factor to the guilt experienced by these men. Attendance at the birth is an expectation of involved parenting, and expectant fathers often feel coercion to be present in the delivery from healthcare providers, partners, family, and friends (Johnson, 2002).

Consistent with other studies, the prominence of the provider role was central to these fathers. Premberg et al. (2008) noted that to become a father meant to gain a new responsibility, including giving the child a secure upbringing and providing for a family. Similarly, the fathers in this study were more aware of their vulnerability, avoided risky situations, and took precautions for their own safety.

Fatherhood carries culturally prescribed behavioral requirements and consensus regarding paternal role expectations (Knoester et al., 2007). Primarily, men are expected to be engaged, accessible, and responsible fathers (Lamb, 2003). Despite the extended geographic separation of the men in this study, they attempted to fulfill this role through online and telephone communication with their spouses. Not only did frequent communication allay some of the psychological distress they experienced because of their absence, but it also helped to restore balance to the protector and provider role. The men extolled the merits of communication with their spouses—primarily that it gave them a sense of being there and made them feel like involved and contributing partners.

The impact of maternal influence on fathering behaviors and attitudes is an area of evolving research. Jordan (1990) stressed the importance of a supportive context as crucial to the new father's development and noted that the recognition that a father received served to promote or to hinder his role development. In corroborating studies, the salience of the mother's role has been demonstrated in defining and shaping the paternal role. Sharing information about infants' daily events and developmental progress while fathers were working outside the home helped working fathers get to know their infants better (Barclay & Lupton, 1999). Mothers provided emotional support by encouraging fathers' involvement with their infant (Goodman, 2005). Clearly, the men in this study felt a connection to their newborns that was achieved through communication with their wives. Whether this connection then translates to increased paternal involvement and sharing of childcare duties remains to be seen. Father involvement has positive consequences for children's development (Pleck & Masciadrelli, 2004), so it is hoped that this early and frequent communication facilitates paternal role transition and sets the stage for a favorable father–child relationship.

Limitations

Although the first-time fathers who participated in this study reflected the diversity of the military in terms of ethnicity, age, and education, each of the men belonged to a traditional nuclear family. This study was not focused on different kinds of families, despite the many family types

Nursing Research   January/February 2010 Vol 59, No 1

that exist. In addition, the experiences of these new fathers are examined within an ethnocentric view of fatherhood common in Western countries; all new and expectant fathers may not hold the same expectations of their role. The results cannot be generalized beyond the participants in this study because lived experiences differ for individuals according to context and time. Instead, these findings may be used to contribute to theory development and practice. Lastly, the interviews were conducted 2 to 6 months after the children were born; thus, the possibility exists that the recall of events and feelings was diminished through time delay.

Conclusions

Few men make the transition to fatherhood under intense conditions of both a combat environment and a geographic separation from their spouse. The stories of these 17 men help to understand the fears and the anxieties they experienced as well as the ameliorative effects of communication with their spouses. Communication between partners in this study served to alleviate some of the men's psychological distress and promoted a connection with their newborns.

The relevance of these findings is not limited to combat military nurses. Understanding new fathers' experiences and perspectives assists nurses in identifying better ways to prepare and to support men in an involved fatherhood role, despite the limitations of a stressful combat environment and geographic separation. This information can be used to set the stage for healthy reunions, which may take place at military bases and within communities across the globe, and thus is of benefit to all nurses working with military families. ◼

Accepted for publication August 17 2009.

The author thanks Dr. Linda Grimsley (Albany State University) for her guidance and editorial contributions.

Corresponding author: Kathleen A. Schachman, PhD, APRN-BC, Montana State University, Bozeman, MT 59717 (e-mail: Kathleen. schachman@montana.edu).

References

Barclay, L., & Lupton, D. (1999). The experiences of new fatherhood: A socio-cultural analysis. *Journal of Advanced Nursing, 29*(4), 1013–1020.

Colaizzi, P. (1978). Psychological research as the phenomenologist views it. In R. Valle & M. King (Eds.), *Existential-phenomenological alternatives for psychology* (pp. 48–71). New York: Oxford University Press.

Deave, T., & Johnson, D. (2008). The transition to parenthood: What does it mean for fathers? *Journal of Advanced Nursing, 63*(6), 626–633.

Department of Defense, Statistical Information Analysis Division. (2009). *Active duty military personnel strengths by region and country.* Retrieved April 1, 2009, from http://siadapp.dmdc. osd.mil/personnel/MILITARY/history/hst0812.pdf

Draper, J. (2003). Men's passage to fatherhood: An analysis of the contemporary relevance of transition theory. *Nursing Inquiry, 10*(1), 66–77.

Essex, H. N., & Pickett, K. E. (2008). Mothers without companionship during childbirth: An analysis within the Millennium Cohort Study. *Birth, 35*(4), 266–276.

Goodman, J. H. (2005). Becoming an involved father of an infant. *Journal of Obstetric, Gynecologic and Neonatal Nursing, 34*(2), 190–200.

Hodnett, E. D., Gates, S., Hofmeyer, G. J., & Sakala, C. (2007). Continuous support for women during childbirth. *Cochrane Database of Systematic Reviews, 3*(CD003766).

Johnson, M. P. (2002). An exploration of men's experience and role at childbirth. *Journal of Men's Studies, 11*(1), 165–182.

Jordan, P. L. (1990). Laboring for relevance: Expectant and new fatherhood. *Nursing Research, 39*(1), 11–16.

Knoester, C., Petts, R. J., & Eggebeen, D. J. (2007). Commitments to fathering and the well-being and social participation of new, disadvantaged fathers. *Journal of Marriage and the Family, 69*(4), 991–1004.

Lamb, M. E. (2003). *The role of the father in child development* (4th ed.). Hoboken, NJ: Wiley.

Pleck, J. H., & Masciadrelli, B. P. (2004). Paternal involvement by U.S. residential fathers: Levels, sources, and consequences. In M. E. Lamb (Ed.), *The role of the father in child development* (4th ed., pp. 222–271). Hoboken, NJ: Wiley.

Premberg, A., Hellstrom, A. L., & Berg, M. (2008). Experiences of the first year as father. *Scandinavian Journal of Caring Sciences, 22*(1), 56–63.

Reed, R. K. (2005). *Birthing fathers: The transformation of men in American rites of birth.* Piscataway, NJ: Rutgers University Press.

Rosich-Medina, A., & Shetty, A. (2007). Paternal experiences of pregnancy and labour. *British Journal of Midwifery, 15*(2), 66–70.

Streubert, H. J., & Carpenter, D. R. (1999). *Qualitative research in nursing: Advancing the humanistic imperative* (2nd ed.). Philadelphia: Lippincott.